Kallmann Syndrome and Hypogonadotropic Hypogonadism

Frontiers of Hormone Research

Vol. 39

Series Editor

Ashley B. Grossman London

Kallmann Syndrome and Hypogonadotropic Hypogonadism

Volume Editor

Richard Quinton Newcastle-upon-Tyne

20 figures, 5 in color, and 12 tables, 2010

KARGER

Basel · Freiburg · Paris · London · New York · Bangalore ·
Bangkok · Shanghai · Singapore · Tokyo · Sydney

Richard Quinton, MA, MD, FRCP
Endocrine Research Group
Institute of Human Genetics
University of Newcastle-upon-Tyne
Newcastle-upon-Tyne
United Kingdom

Library of Congress Cataloging-in-Publication Data

Kallmann syndrome and hypogonadotropic hypogonadism / volume editor, Richard Quinton.
p. ; cm. – (Frontiers of hormone research, ISSN 0301–3073 ; vol. 39)
Includes bibliographical references and indexes.
ISBN 978–3–8055–8617–7 (hard cover: alk. paper)
1. Hypogonadism. I. Quinton, Richard. II. Series: Frontiers of hormone research,
v. 39. 0301–3073 ;
[DNLM: 1. Hypogonadism–genetics. 2. Kallmann Syndrome–genetics.
W1 FR946F v.39 2010 / WK 900 K14 2010]
RC898.K35 2010
616.4′7–dc22

2010006846

Bibliographic Indices. This publication is listed in bibliographic services, including Current Contents® and PubMed/MEDLINE.

Disclaimer. The statements, opinions and data contained in this publication are solely those of the individual authors and contributors and not of the publisher and the editor(s). The appearance of advertisements in the book is not a warranty, endorsement, or approval of the products or services advertised or of their effectiveness, quality or safety. The publisher and the editor(s) disclaim responsibility for any injury to persons or property resulting from any ideas, methods, instructions or products referred to in the content or advertisements.

Drug Dosage. The authors and the publisher have exerted every effort to ensure that drug selection and dosage set forth in this text are in accord with current recommendations and practice at the time of publication. However, in view of ongoing research, changes in government regulations, and the constant flow of information relating to drug therapy and drug reactions, the reader is urged to check the package insert for each drug for any change in indications and dosage and for added warnings and precautions. This is particularly important when the recommended agent is a new and/or infrequently employed drug.

www.karger.com
Printed in Switzerland on acid-free and non-aging paper (ISO 9706) by Reinhardt Druck, Basel
ISSN 0301–3073
ISBN 978–3–8055–8617–7
e-ISBN 978–3–8055–8618–4

Contents

Foreword

One of the major clinical advances in neuroendocrinology over the past decade has been the increasing understanding of the processes of regulation of gonadotropin-releasing hormone and its dysfunction in a clinical setting. As new regulatory peptides have been identified, the underlying causes of central hypogonadism have multiplied and the area has become increasingly complex. The reversibility of even genetically determined hypogonadotropic hypogonadism has become more firmly established, and once again clinical studies, of what used to be called 'sports of nature', have greatly expanded our understanding of basic physiological pathways. This is now an excellent point at which to take stock of the most recent progress, to put it into some form of structure, and to aid scientists and clinicians in getting to grips with this mass of new knowledge in planning future research and in treating our patients. Richard Quinton has put together a stellar group of experts in this area, and has provided a comprehensive overview of this burgeoning field. This is an excellent starting point for those caring for patients with delayed puberty, hypogonadotropic hypogonadism and other forms of central reproductive disorder, and I hope will stimulate others to work in this area.

Ashley B. Grossman, London

Preface

When I joined the research team of my friend and mentor Dr (now Professor) Pierre Bouloux back in the early 1990s, a number of things seemed evident to myself and many other investigators at the time [1]. Analysis of the relatively small number of published idiopathic hypogonadotropic hypogonadism (IHH) kindreds had long defined three mendelian modes of inheritance, X-linked recessive, autosomal dominant and autosomal recessive, so it seemed reasonable to infer the existence of at least three genes. However, nobody anticipated that the number would ever run into double figures. *GNRH1* was the original candidate gene for normosmic IHH, but no mutations were found in the small (by present day standards) number of patient DNAs expensively and laboriously sequenced. *GNRHR* did not seem to be a promising candidate, due to the near-universal responsiveness of IHH patients to exogenous GnRH pulses. *KAL1*, the very first IHH-related gene had just been discovered, and so it seemed that a predominantly X-linked mode of disease inheritance and/or the occurrence of de novo *KAL1* germline mutations constituted a possible explanation for the observed male preponderance of cases (which, in fact, remains unexplained to this day).

The extracranial origin of GnRH neurons in the olfactory placode and their migration into the forebrain along fibres of the olfactory and (in mammals) the accessory olfactory nerves had also just been discovered. Moreover, a striking migration defect was observed in a single Xpter-deleted fetus from an X-linked Kallmann syndrome (KS) kindred. This elegant model of arrested GnRH neuron migration was assumed to underpin all forms of KS and, possibly, also of normosmic IHH (where perhaps migration arrest occurred through a mechanism independent of olfactory fibre misguidance). One consequence of universalising this model was to draw a clear line of separation between syndromic IHH and the 'functional' forms of gonadotropin deficiency that occur in relation to simple pubertal delay (like IHH, far more common in males), weight loss and stress (typically observed as hypothalamic amenorrhoea in women) and during episodes of acute illness or chronic disease. Unlike these time-limited perturbations of the GnRH pulse generator, syndromic IHH was considered to be a lifelong irreversible condition. Another was to see IHH as being entirely distinct from the primary pituitary gonadotropin deficiency observed in some syndromic forms of combined pituitary hormone deficiency.

Thinking back over these ideas and concepts, the cautionary lyrics of a famous Blues artist come to mind: 'It ain't necessarily so...'

In many of their research grant applications, researchers in the field of IHH, including KS – its anosmic form, will have referred to how the study of this rare disease model has the potential to illuminate the processes behind normal human embryonic development and postnatal pubertal maturation. For all the truth in this statement, I suspect that many of us would admit to our primary drive being fascination with the manifestations and biological basis of IHH itself. Nevertheless, as evidenced by the following chapters from a remarkable group of contributors across the globe, it is now increasingly clear that each of the different genetic mechanisms by which IHH is caused represents a small but defined point of vulnerability to human reproductive success.

What are the evolutionary pressures that have maintained these heterozygous IHH-predisposing alleles circulating among present day human populations, such that full-blown IHH can occur in those individuals whose inherited burden of genetic defects is sufficient to critically impair neuroendocrine control of reproduction? In mammals, the capacity to grow and reproduce is intimately linked to the nutritional status. It is thus tempting to speculate that ancestral exposure to periods of sickness or famine, when it would have been counterproductive to invest scarce energy resources into reproduction and ensuing childcare, has left an imprint on our genetic lineage – of which cases of IHH may represent a tangible echo.

Finally, on behalf of myself and other investigators, I would like to offer my thanks and appreciation to those IHH patients who have allowed us into their families, as it were, to undertake detailed phenotyping and genetic analysis. Many of these individuals have experienced challenging physical and emotional lives before coming under the care of an informed and sympathetic physician or establishing contact with a patient support group. Their stories, questions and concerns can be found at www.kallmanns.org, so I will leave the final say to Neil Smith, one of its founder members:

'My own experience of having KS and from talking to others with KS and IHH is that there is a real advantage to knowing the genetic cause behind the condition. There is an almost cathartic experience in being able to pin-point the cause of one's condition, rather than the more common patient experience of being told 'it just happens'. While participation in genetic studies may have no impact on current treatment, I always encourage fellow patients to take part in the hope that they can find a reason for their own condition and possibly help future generations of patients. In the not too distant future, we look forward to being able to get a rapid read-out from our DNA samples on an 'IHH/Kallmann gene chip'.'

Richard Quinton, Newcastle-upon-Tyne

Reference

1 Bouloux PM, Munroe P, Kirk JM, Besser GM: Sex and smell – an enigma resolved. J Endocrinol 1992;133:323–326.

Quinton R (ed): Kallmann Syndrome and Hypogonadotropic Hypogonadism.
Front Horm Res. Basel, Karger, 2010, vol 39, pp 1–12

Molecular Characterization and Phenotypic Expression of Mutations in Genes for Gonadotropins and Their Receptors in Humans

Roberto Salvi · François P. Pralong

Service of Endocrinology, Diabetology and Metabolism, University Hospital, Lausanne, Switzerland

Abstract

Gonadotropin hormones undergo important dynamic changes during life. Their rise during puberty stimulates gonadal steroid secretion, triggering the development of secondary sexual characteristics and the acquisition of fertility. The full spectrum of possible mutations and polymorphisms in the human gonadotropins and in their receptor genes has been described in recent years. Patients harboring these mutations display a very wide range of phenotypes affecting all aspects of the reproductive axis. An important insight provided by the careful study of these patients lies in the striking gender differences in the phenotypes associated with a given mutation. As a result, the careful study of these rare patients has allowed us to better define the respective roles of luteinizing hormone and follicle-stimulating hormone in normal human pubertal development and in the achievement of full fertility potential in either males or females. In this work, we describe briefly the known mutations in the genes for both gonadotropins and their receptors, and discuss their genotype/phenotype correlations in light of these important gender differences.

The hormones of the human reproductive axis undergo important dynamic changes during life. In the fetal and neonatal periods, gonadotropins are secreted at levels similar to those seen in early puberty, but their levels then fall close to the assay detection thresholds during infancy until pubertal development begins. This neonatal 'minipuberty' is particularly pronounced in boys, though due to the absence of androgen receptors on Sertoli cells, spermatogenesis does not occur at this stage [1]. The onset of puberty results from the stimulation of gonadal steroid secretion, corresponding to the appearance and development of secondary sexual characteristics and, eventually, the acquisition of the full fertility potential of normal adults.

Activity of the gonadotropic axis is then largely maintained throughout adult life. The delicate sequence of events characterizing normal reproductive activity in all mammals is critically dependent upon the activity of the hypothalamic gonadotropin-releasing hormone (GnRH): a pulsatile secretion of GnRH into vessels of the hypothalamo-pituitary portal system is mandatory to induce the synthesis and release of the two gonadotropins, luteinizing hormone (LH) and follicle-stimulating hormone (FSH), by gonadotroph cells of the anterior pituitary gland [2]. In general terms, LH secreted in the periphery will stimulate gonadal steroid biosynthesis and secretion, whereas FSH regulates gametogenesis in both men and women. However, new insights into the physiological regulation of the gonadotropic axis in humans have been gained by the careful phenotyping of individuals bearing mutations of genes acting at different levels of the axis [3–5].

Indeed, the full spectrum of possible mutations and polymorphisms in the genes encoding human gonadotropins and their receptors has been described in recent years. Both gain-of-function and loss-of-function mutations have been reported in the receptors for LH (LH-R) and FSH (FSH-R). Although gain-of-function mutations remain exceptional, the loss-of-function mutations are associated with various phenotypic forms of hypergonadotropic hypogonadism [6]. With respect to the gonadotropins themselves, mutations in the β-subunit genes of either LH or FSH are associated with the few cases of isolated gonadotropin deficiency known to date [7–13]. The genetics and phenotypes associated with the various known mutations of the human gonadotropins and their receptors are described below.

Gonadotropins

The two gonadotropins LH and FSH are heterodimeric hormones composed of a common α-subunit and a specific β-subunit. Both hormones belong to the superfamily of cysteine knot growth factors that also comprises transforming growth factor-β, nerve growth factor and platelet-derived growth factor. This classification results from striking similarities in protein tertiary, rather than in their primary amino-acid sequence [14]. One of the important characteristics of this superfamily is the existence of three cysteine disulfide bonds in each of these two subunits. A key component of the cysteine knot motif is an eight-amino acid ring that contains two of the disulphide bonds and which is penetrated by the third bond. Central to the formation of the eight-amino acid ring in all human glycoprotein hormone β-subunits is the sequence CAGYC. The conserved glycine is crucial to avoid steric hindrance of the third, ring-penetrating disulphide bond. This somewhat complicated structure, where both subunits are associated via a so-called 'seat-belt', bears an important functional role for glycoprotein hormones [15, 16], indispensable for proper receptor binding and activation. A number of mutations in the β-subunit genes of both gonadotropins have been described (fig. 1).

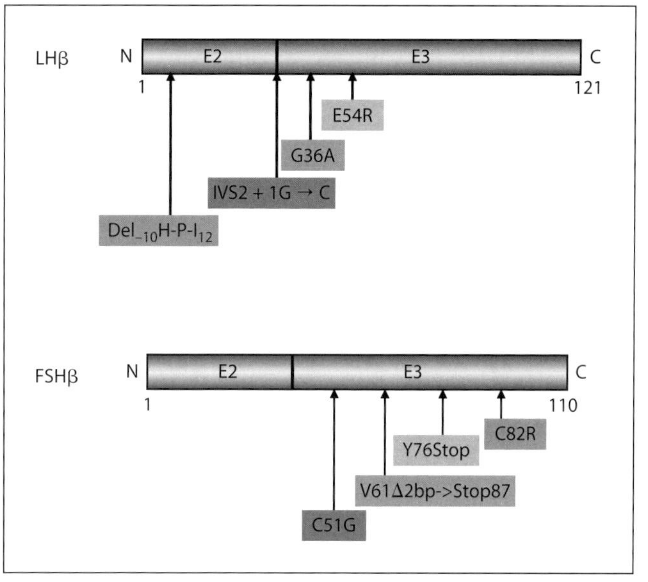

Fig. 1. Schematic representations of the currently known inactivating mutations in the LHβ and FSHβ subunit proteins.

Luteinizing Hormone, the LHβ Subunit

Five men and 2 women with a mutation in *LHB*, the gene encoding LHβ have been described [10–13], one of the men in a collaboration between the group of A. Beckers and our laboratory [11], with the woman and 2 of the other men belonging to the same nuclear family [12]. The 5 men had a very similar phenotype and, notably, were normally masculinized at birth. The most recently described case was, however, exceptional in having near-normal size testes and qualitatively and quantitatively normal spermatogenesis [13]. Nevertheless, these five observations concur to demonstrate that LH is not necessary for fetal male gender differentiation, for which a primary role for placental chorionic gonadotropin (hCG) in stimulating fetal Leydig cells can be inferred. These men also all presented with an absence of spontaneous puberty, confirming the crucial importance of pituitary LH for normal pubertal development and acquisition of secondary sexual characteristics. In contrast, the only 2 females known to date with an inactivating mutation of *LHB* had normal pubertal development; normal thelarche and adrenarche, but later developed secondary amenorrhea with infertility [12, 13]. These observations demonstrate that FSH alone is sufficient to elicit secretion of sufficient estrogen to permit the acquisition of secondary sexual characteristics in human females, even in the absence of LH. However, in the absence of LH stimulation, the amount of estrogens produced probably remains very low, there is no follicular growth beyond the early antral stage, and ovulation does not occur. Sonography instead shows ovarian macrocysts.

Despite the broadly similar clinical phenotypes of the male patients known to bear an inactivating mutation of *LHB*, they had strikingly different genotypic abnormalities.

The first patient [10], initially described by Axelrod et al. [17], presented as a 17-year-old boy with delayed puberty, elevated LH and FSH, and undetectable serum testosterone. On testicular biopsy, no Leydig cells were seen, and spermatogenesis was halted. This patient harbored a homozygous missense mutation of the LHβ gene, inducing a glutamine to arginine substitution at position 54. This substitution was shown by the authors to prevent LH binding to its receptor, but did not alter heterodimerization between the α- and β-subunits. Thus, immunogenicity of LH was preserved, and hormone levels were detectable and above the normal range due to absent negative sex steroid feedback.

The patient that we subsequently described harbored a homozygous missense mutation inducing a glycine to aspartate amino acid substitution at position 36 of the LHβ subunit [11]. Because this amino acid substitution involved the CAGYC region of the subunit, it was found to abolish heterodimeric LH formation. As a result, we could not measure any circulating LH in this patient who presented with isolated LH deficiency. This is consistent with previous reports showing that free LHβ subunits are inefficiently secreted in vitro, and that dimerization with the glycoprotein α-subunit is required to permit secretion of LH [18, 19]. Thus, in our patient, the absence of circulating intact LH and free LHβ was probably due to the prevention of LH dimerization and secretion by the mutated LHβ subunit.

Another homozygous mutation described recently in a consanguineous family with 3 affected siblings abolished a 5′ splice site, thus interfering in a major way both with processing of *LHB* mRNA and with heterodimerization of LH, resulting in impaired LH secretion [12].

Most recently, a homozygous 9bp deletion in exon 2 that resulted in deletion of amino acid residues 10–12 was identified in a consanguineous Moroccan family. The shortened LHβ subunit was only slightly less efficient at heterodimerizing than wild type, and the resulting LH heterodimer was, in turn, of only slightly reduced bioactivity. Moreover, LH-mediated intratesticular testosterone levels were relatively preserved – factors that may in part explain the normal spermatogenesis. However, extragonadal circulating LH and testosterone levels were low (LH <0.05 IU/l). The reason for this was hypothesized to lie in decreased stability of the mutant protein and/or reduced stability or translational efficiency of its corresponding mRNA.

Thus, although the external phenotypes of patients harboring *LHβ* subunit mutations may be very similar, circulating LH levels may be high, low or undetectable, depending on the nature of the mutation, giving an appearance of either hyper- or hypogonadotropic hypogonadism.

Follicle-Stimulating Hormone, the FSHβ Subunit

A total of 3 men and 4 women with an inactivating *FSHβ* mutation have been reported. In contrast to isolated LH deficiency in males [11, 17], 2 of the reported men presented with primary infertility after completion of a clinically normal puberty [7, 8]. They were both normally virilized, and had normal serum levels of testosterone in the face of slightly elevated LH levels, consistent with a primary role for LH rather than FSH in the stimulation of testosterone production and secretion during normal puberty. However, the testicular volume of both of these men was small, and they also had low or undetectable levels of serum FSH.

The phenotype of the 3rd affected male reported in the literature is more puzzling, since this man presented at age 18 years with delayed puberty [9]. On physical exam, he looked prepubertal with no axillary or facial hair, and had small testis bilaterally. His laboratory workup disclosed a relatively high serum LH of 24.5 IU/l, low testosterone levels and undetectable FSH. This phenotype is somewhat peculiar, because Leydig cells do not normally express the FSH receptor, and should therefore respond to LH stimulation even in the absence of FSH. It has therefore been hypothesized that hyporesponsiveness of the Leydig cells in this particular patient resulted from the lack of a local factor whose production is FSH dependent [9]. Thus, the phenotypic differences between the 3 male patients with *FSHβ* mutations may relate to differences in the severity of the mutation.

Genotype-phenotype correlations point towards amino acids 61–76 of the *FSHβ* sequence as important determinants of severity of phenotype [20], but the hypothesis could not be confirmed in vitro, since no differences were noted between all known mutations of the *FSHβ* genes [20]. This question therefore remains open, and it could be speculated that delayed puberty in the patient reported by Philipp et al. [9] resulted from other unidentified defect(s) [3]. Regardless of these differences, all 3 male patients with isolated FSH deficiency were completely azoospermic, which would suggest a crucial role for FSH in spermatogenesis. These data are however in contrast to the observations made in men with inactivating *FSH-R* mutations, who had variable degrees of oligozoospermia (see below). The true role of FSH in spermatogenesis therefore remains somewhat open to question until more patients can be studied.

In contrast to men, women with *FSHβ* mutations all share the similar phenotype of primary amenorrhea, partial breast development and infertility [7, 20–22]. On laboratory workup, they typically have low levels of circulating estradiol and progesterone; their LH levels are high, and FSH undetectable. Interestingly, the 2 male patients described above with a mutation in the *FSHβ* gene who underwent normal pubertal development had sisters affected by the same mutation, and these sisters shared the female phenotype of primary amenorrhea generally described. There seems thus to be a gender difference in the phenotypic expression of inactivating mutations in *FSHβ*.

Gonadotropin Receptors

As is the case for their ligands, the two gonadotropin receptors LH-R and FSH-R are structurally highly related molecules that belong to a subfamily within the G-protein-coupled receptor superfamily [23]. This subfamily also includes the receptor for the

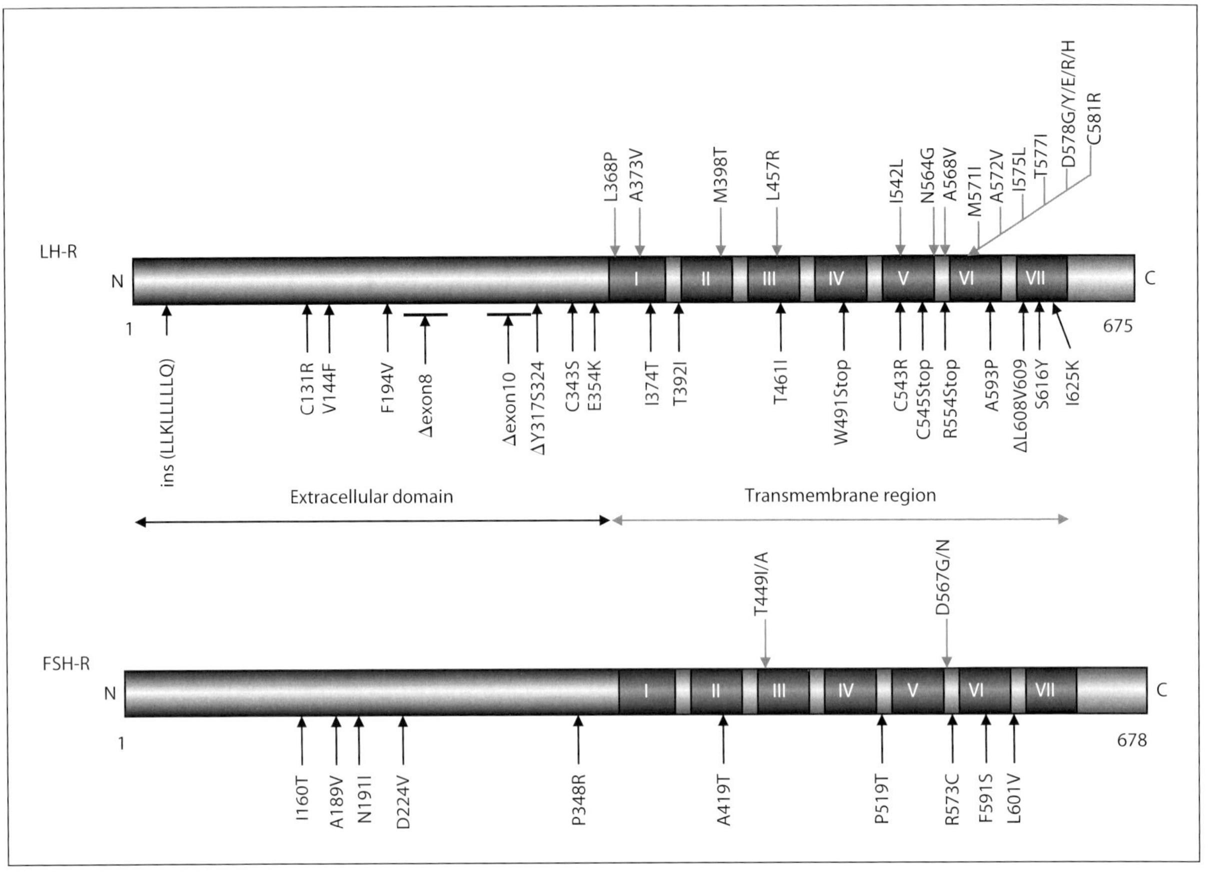

Fig. 2. Schematic representations of the currently known mutations in the mature LH-R and FSH-R proteins. Inactivating mutations are indicated with black arrows/lines and activating mutations with grey arrows/lines. Most original descriptions can be found in references [3, 37, 38].

other glycoprotein hormone TSH. It is characterized by an unusually large N-terminal extra cellular ligand-binding domain containing several leucine-rich repeats, in addition to the rhodopsin-like seven-transmembrane helices. The third and last domain of these receptors consists of a relatively short intracellular C-terminal tail. Both the *LH-R* and *FSH-R* genes have a similar organization, and are located in different portions of the short arm of chromosome 2 (2p21 and 2p21-16, respectively). The high sequence homology and the close genomic localization between the two gonadotropin receptors reminds us that they arose through gene duplication, followed by functional divergence.

Mutations affecting the gonadotropin receptors contrast with those affecting their ligands in two key areas (fig. 2): first, both gain-of-function and loss-of-function mutations have been reported, and second, loss-of-function mutations are invariably associated with hypergonadotropic hypogonadism.

Luteinizing Hormone Receptor

Human *LH-R* gene spans ~70 kb and consists of 11 exons separated by 10 introns. It is also referred to as *LHCG-R*, since it is also the receptor for hCG. The first 10 exons encode the large extracellular portion of the cell-surface receptor, with exon 11 encoding both the seven-transmembrane and C-terminal intracellular domains [24]. Very recently, an additional exon located between exon 6 and exon 7 has been discovered. This novel exon 6A obviously does not code for the final/mature receptor protein, but appears to have a regulatory function at the level of gene transcription [25]. LH-R is predominantly expressed in the gonads; in the testes, expression is mainly restricted to Leydig cells, but in the ovary, expression occurs in differentiated granulosa cells, theca cells, interstitial and luteal cells. Extragonadal LH-R expression has also been detected in several tissues, including uterus, fallopian tubes, placenta, brain and lymphocytes. However, physiological relevance of receptor expression in nongonadal tissues is not supported by clinical observations in individuals with either activating or inactivating mutations of the *LH-R* gene.

In addition to the main transcript coding for the full-length protein, thee other splice variants have been shown to be transcribed from the human *LH-R* gene in gonadal tissues, although proof that these are translated into the corresponding polypeptides is lacking. Translation of the full-length mRNA gives rise to a single polypeptide chain of 699 residues, including the 24-residue-long signal peptide that is subsequently removed during intracellular processing. The mature LH-R is therefore composed of 675 residues with a predicted molecular mass of 75 kDa, but without taking into account that this receptor is a glycoprotein. In fact, transfection experiments in mammalian cell lines have shown that an 85- to 95-kDa band detected on SDS-PAGE is the mature glycosylated LH-R present at the cell surface. This mature form arises from the maturation and transport of a 68- to 75-kDa precursor glycoprotein that is localized in the endoplasmic reticulum. The extracellular domain of the receptor has 340 amino acids and contains six N-linked glycosylation sites. This is followed by a region containing the seven membrane-spanning segments interconnected by three extracellular and three intracellular loops. Then the receptor ends with a relatively short C-terminal intracellular tail.

The extracellular domain is responsible for binding to the LH and CG ligands with high affinity. The three-dimensional structure of LH-R has not yet been determined, but recent data published on the crystallographic structure of the FSH bound to the extracellular domain of FSH-R are illuminating in this regard [26], giving the structural relatedness between the two gonadotropin receptors. LH-R mediates gonadotropin signaling by triggering intracellular responses involved in gonadal maturation and function, as well as regulation of steroidogenesis and gametogenesis. These physiological effects are mainly mediated through the activation of the Gαs/adenyl cyclase/cAMP/PKA pathway. The cascade of these signaling events eventually results in the synthesis of the sex steroids testosterone, estradiol and progesterone. Activation of inositol phosphate and MAPK pathways has also been reported, although their relative importance in normal and clinical settings has still to be fully determined.

Activating *LH-R* mutations result in gonadotropin-independent, male-limited precocious puberty [27]. The observation that the same mutation did not induce any phenotype in female carriers is consistent with the hypothesis that in the ovary, LH-R expression is triggered by FSH priming. Therefore, no expression of the mutated receptor can occur before the normal start of puberty in females. Interestingly, loss-of-function mutations in the LH-R also exhibit a gender-dependent phenotypic expression: female patients usually have hypergonadotropic hypogonadism associated with normal secondary sexual characteristics [6], whereas male patients present with a variable degree of genital ambiguity depending on the degree of functional impairment of the receptor [6, 28]. The exceptional case of a patient with an LH receptor mutation presenting as delayed puberty and azoospermia was also reported [29]. The normal sexual differentiation and the appropriate response of testosterone to hCG stimulation in this patient in whom a large part of exon 10 of the LH receptor was deleted resulted from a differential activation of the receptor by LH and hCG [30]. Taken together, all these reports demonstrate the physiological importance of the LH-LH receptor system for normal sex differentiation and spermatogenesis in the male, and for fertility in the female.

Follicle-Stimulating Hormone Receptor

The human *FSH-R* gene spans 54 kb of genomic DNA and is composed of 10 exons interspersed with 9 introns, with the last exon coding for the seven-transmembrane and intracellular domains, while all the other exons encode the large extracellular domain [31]. It has been speculated that during evolution, the ancestral *FSH-R* gene (as well as *TSH-R*) lost its final intron, analogous to the one still present in the *LH-R* gene, resulting in the current arrangement of 10 exons and 9 introns. In contrast to the expression pattern of LH-R, FSH-R expression is strictly gonadic and highly cell-specific. Expression is confined on Sertoli cells in testes and on granulosa cells in the ovary.

The FSH-R is a single polypeptide composed of 695 residues, including the first 17 residues which encode a hydrophobic signal peptide. Mature, glycosylated, recombinant FSH-R is a protein of approximately 80 kDa. The extracellular ligand-binding domain of the receptor has 359 residues and contains four N-linked glycosylation sites. Glycosylation does not seem to be required for ligand binding, but rather for proper folding and trafficking of the receptor to the membrane. Recently, the determination of the three-dimensional structure of human FSH complexed with the extracellular binding-domain of its receptor has been accomplished. Accordingly, the extracellular domain of the FSH-R is shaped as a slightly curved tube, and the FSH hormone binds to the inner, slightly concave face of the tube in a hand-clasp fashion [26]. This model may have implications for the LH/

LH-R interactions, since it has been suggested that all glycoprotein hormones bind to their receptors in this mode, and that binding specificity is mediated by key interaction sites involving both the common α- and hormone specific β-subunits. Signaling transduction of FSH-R is analogous to that of LH-R, in that ligand binding is followed by cAMP increase through the activation of the Gαs/adenyl cyclase/cAMP/PKA pathway, ultimately leading to sex steroid synthesis in either Sertoli or granulosa cells.

The only known activating FSH-R mutation was identified in a male patient. He underwent hypophysectomy for pituitary adenoma, and spermatogenesis was found to persist after surgery despite undetectable levels of gonadotropins [32]. No spontaneously activating mutation of the FSH-R has been described in a woman yet, although FSH-R mutations have been identified in patients diagnosed with pregnancy-associated ovarian hyperstimulation syndrome [27]. In these patients, the mutation introduces a conformational change in the receptor, rendering it susceptible to stimulation by the high levels of hCG occurring during pregnancy.

As is the case for the LH-R, a gender-specific expression of loss-of-function mutations is observed with the FSH-R. The first missense mutation of the FSH receptor, located in the extracellular domain of the protein and leading to impaired cell surface expression, was initially reported in hypergonadotropic hypogonadic Finnish women presenting with primary amenorrhea and a variable degree of delayed pubertal development [33]. Ovarian dysgenesis was found in many of these women, but some degree of follicular maturation was nevertheless observed in others [33]. Five male family members homozygous for the same mutation were subsequently identified [34]: they were all normally virilized and had normal testosterone levels with high FSH and normal or high LH levels. Surprisingly, azoospermia was not the rule, some of these men exhibiting only a moderate degree of teratozoospermia. Two of these patients had even fathered 2 children.

These findings challenge the concept of FSH being the critical hormone for human spermatogenesis, especially since they almost exactly corroborate the phenotype observed in mice deficient for either FSH-β or the FSH-R [35, 36]. However, FSH is clearly crucial for normal follicular development in human females [37]. In males, FSH may not constitute an absolute requirement for the initiation and maintenance of spermatogenesis, but it is needed for optimal sperm production. However, the hypothesis that mutations in the FSH receptor could be widely responsible for the syndrome of 'idiopathic' male infertility could not be confirmed [38].

Conclusions

The identification of a wide range of mutations in the genes encoding the two gonadotropins, LH and FSH, and their respective receptors has provided invaluable insight into their physiological role in gender determination, pubertal development and the acquisition of a full fertility potential. These various observations have also raised important issues that remain unresolved. One of these relates to the precise relative importance of each gonadotropin hormone for the pubertal development of either male or female subjects. For example, inactivation of the LHβ gene results in secondary amenorrhea and infertility, whereas LH-R mutations have no phenotype in the affected females. An even more puzzling discrepancy is found between different male patients affected by inactivating mutations in the *FSHB* gene, where 2 of them exhibited essentially normal pubertal development, whereas a 3rd had delayed puberty despite high-normal LH secretion. These examples illustrate both the power of such genotype-phenotype correlations, as well as their limitations when patient numbers are small, underlying the need to pursue the phenotypic characterization of these rare patients when they present to us.

References

1 Boukari K, Meduri G, Brailly-Tabard S, Guibourdenche J, Ciampi ML, Massin N, Martinerie L, Picard JY, Rey R, Lombès M, Young J: Lack of androgen receptor expression in Sertoli cells accounts for the absence of anti-Mullerian hormone repression during early human testis development. J Clin Endocrinol Metab 2009;94:1818–1825.

2 Marshall JC, Kelch RP: Gonadotropin-releasing hormone: role of pulsatile secretion in the regulation of reproduction. N Engl J Med 1986;315:1459–1468.

3 Huhtaniemi IT, Themmen AP: Mutations in human gonadotropin and gonadotropin-receptor genes. Endocrine 2005;26:207–217.

4 Pralong FP: Genetic basis of hypothalamic-pituitary hypogonadism; in Rappaport R (ed): Hypothalamic-Pituitary Development. Genetic and Clinical Aspects. Basel, Karger, 2001, pp 122–139.

5 Trarbach EB, Silveira LG, Latronico AC: Genetic insights into human isolated gonadotropin deficiency. Pituitary 2007;10:381–391.

6 Beck-Peccoz P, Romoli R, Persani L: Mutations of LH and FSH receptors. J Endocrinol Invest 2000;23: 566–572.

7 Layman LC, Lee EJ, Peak DB, Namnoum AB, Vu KV, van Lingen BL, Gray MR, McDonough PG, Reindollar RH, Jameson JL: Delayed puberty and hypogonadism caused by mutations in the follicle-stimulating hormone beta-subunit gene. N Engl J Med 1997;337:607–611.

8 Lindstedt G, Nystrom E, Matthews C, Ernest I, Janson PO, Chatterjee VK: Follitropin (FSH) deficiency in an infertile male due to FSHbeta gene mutation. A syndrome of normal puberty and virilization but underdeveloped testicles with azoospermia, low FSH but high lutropin and normal serum testosterone concentrations. Clin Chem Lab Med 1998;36:663–665.

9 Phillip M, Arbelle JE, Segev Y, Parvari R: Male hypogonadism due to a mutation in the gene for the beta-subunit of follicle-stimulating hormone. N Engl J Med 1998;338:1729–1732.

10 Weiss J, Axelrod L, Whitcomb RW, Harris PE, Crowley WF, Jameson JL: Hypogonadism caused by a single amino acid substitution in the beta subunit of luteinizing hormone. N Engl J Med 1992;326:179–183.

11 Valdes-Socin H, Salvi R, Daly AF, Gaillard RC, Quatresooz P, Tebeu PM, Pralong FP, Beckers A: Hypogonadism in a patient with a mutation in the luteinizing hormone beta-subunit gene. N Engl J Med 2004;351:2619–2625.

12 Lofrano-Porto A, Barra GB, Giacomini LA, Nascimento PP, Latronico AC, Casulari LA, da Rocha Neves Fde A: Luteinizing hormone beta mutation and hypogonadism in men and women. N Engl J Med 2007;357:897–904.

13 Achard C, Courtillot C, Lahuna O, Méduri G, Soufir JC, Lière P, Bachelot A, Benyounes H, Schumacher M, Kutenne F, Touraine P, Misrahi M: Normal spermatogenesis in a man with mutant luteinizing hormone. N Engl J Med 2009;361:1856–1863.

14 Vitt UA, Hsu SY, Hsueh AJ: Evolution and classification of cystine knot-containing hormones and related extracellular signaling molecules. Mol Endocrinol 2001;15:681–694.

15 Darling RJ, Wilken JA, Miller-Lindholm AK, Urlacher TM, Ruddon RW, Sherman SA, Bedows E: Functional contributions of noncysteine residues within the cystine knots of human chorionic gonadotropin subunits. J Biol Chem 2001;276:10692–10699.

16 Hayashizaki Y, Hiraoka Y, Endo Y, Miyai K, Matsubara K: Thyroid-stimulating hormone (TSH) deficiency caused by a single base substitution in the CAGYC region of the beta-subunit. EMBO J 1989;8:2291–2296; erratum in EMBO J 1989;8:3542.

17 Axelrod L, Neer RM, Kliman B: Hypogonadism in a male with immunologically active, biologically inactive luteinizing hormone: an exception to a venerable rule. J Clin Endocrinol Metab 1979;48:279–287.

18 Corless CL, Bielinska M, Ramabhadran TV, Daniels-McQueen S, Otani T, Reitz BA, Tiemeier DC, Boime I: Gonadotropin alpha subunit. Differential processing of free and combined forms in human trophoblast and transfected mouse cells. J Biol Chem 1987;262:14197–14203.

19 Matzuk MM, Spangler MM, Camel M, Suganuma N, Boime I: Mutagenesis and chimeric genes define determinants in the beta subunits of human chorionic gonadotropin and lutropin for secretion and assembly. J Cell Biol 1989;109:1429–1438.

20 Layman LC, Porto AL, Xie J, da Motta LA, da Motta LD, Weiser W, Sluss PM: FSH beta gene mutations in a female with partial breast development and a male sibling with normal puberty and azoospermia. J Clin Endocrinol Metab 2002;87:3702–3707.

21 Matthews C, Chatterjee VK: Isolated deficiency of follicle-stimulating hormone re-revisited. N Engl J Med 1997;337:642.

22 Matthews CH, Borgato S, Beck-Peccoz P, Adams M, Tone Y, Gambino G, Casagrande S, Tedeschini G, Benedetti A, Chatterjee VK: Primary amenorrhoea and infertility due to a mutation in the beta-subunit of follicle-stimulating hormone. Nat Genet 1993;5:83–86.

23 Vassart G, Pardo L, Costagliola S: A molecular dissection of the glycoprotein hormone receptors. Trends Biochem Sci 2004;29:119–126.

24 Ascoli M, Fanelli F, Segaloff DL: The lutropin/choriogonadotropin receptor, a 2002 perspective. Endocr Rev 2002;23:141–174.

25 Kossack N, Simoni M, Richter-Unruh A, Themmen AP, Gromoll J: Mutations in a novel, cryptic exon of the luteinizing hormone/chorionic gonadotropin receptor gene cause male pseudohermaphroditism. PLoS Med 2008;5:e88.

26 Fan QR, Hendrickson WA: Structural biology of glycoprotein hormones and their receptors. Endocrine 2005;26:179–188.

27 Huhtaniemi I: Mutations along the pituitary-gonadal axis affecting sexual maturation: novel information from transgenic and knockout mice. Mol Cell Endocrinol 2006;254:84–90.

28 Kremer H, Kraaij R, Toledo SP, Post M, Fridman JB, Hayashida CY, van Reen M, Milgrom E, Ropers HH, Mariman E, Themmen APN, Brunner HG: Male pseudohermaphroditism due to a homozygous missense mutation of the luteinizing hormone receptor gene. Nat Genet 1995;9:160–164.

29 Gromoll J, Eiholzer U, Nieschlag E, Simoni M: Male hypogonadism caused by homozygous deletion of exon 10 of the luteinizing hormone (LH) receptor: differential action of human chorionic gonadotropin and LH. J Clin Endocrinol Metab 2000;85:2281–2286.

30 Muller T, Gromoll J, Simoni M: Absence of exon 10 of the human luteinizing hormone (LH) receptor impairs LH, but not human chorionic gonadotropin action. J Clin Endocrinol Metab 2003;88:2242–2249.

31 Simoni M, Gromoll J, Nieschlag E: The follicle-stimulating hormone receptor: biochemistry, molecular biology, physiology, and pathophysiology. Endocr Rev 1997;18:739–773.

32 Gromoll J, Simoni M, Nieschlag E: An activating mutation of the follicle-stimulating hormone receptor autonomously sustains spermatogenesis in a hypophysectomized man. J Clin Endocrinol Metab 1996;81:1367–1370.

33 Aittomäki K, Lucena JL, Pakarinen P, Sistonen P, Tapanainen J, Gromoll J, Kaskikari R, Sankila EM, Lehväslaiho H, Engel AR, Nieschlag E, Huhtaniemi I, de la Chapelle A: Mutation in the follicle-stimulating hormone receptor gene causes hereditary hypergonadotropic ovarian failure. Cell 1995;82:959–968.

34 Tapanainen JS, Aittomäki K, Min J, Vaskivuo T, Huhtaniemi IT: Men homozygous for an inactivating mutation of the follicle-stimulating hormone (FSH) receptor gene present variable suppression of spermatogenesis and fertility. Nat Genet 1997;15:205–206.

35 Abel MH, Wootton AN, Wilkins V, Huhtaniemi I, Knight PG, Charlton HM: The effect of a null mutation in the follicle-stimulating hormone receptor gene on mouse reproduction. Endocrinology 2000; 141:1795–1803.
36 Kumar TR, Wang Y, Lu N, Matzuk MM: Follicle stimulating hormone is required for ovarian follicle maturation but not male fertility. Nat Genet 1997; 15:201–204.
37 Lussiana C, Guani B, Mari C, Restagno G, Massobrio M, Revelli A: Mutations and polymorphisms of the FSH receptor (FSHR) gene: clinical implications in female fecundity and molecular biology of FSHR protein and gene. Obstet Gynecol Surv 2008;63:785–795.
38 Simoni M, Gromoll J, Höppner W, Kamischke A, Krafft T, Stähle D, Nieschlag E: Mutational analysis of the follicle-stimulating hormone (FSH) receptor in normal and infertile men: identification and characterization of two discrete FSH receptor isoforms. J Clin Endocrinol Metab 1999;84:751–755.

Dr. François P. Pralong
Service of Endocrinology, Diabetology and Metabolism, BH 10-563, University Hospital
Rue du Bugnon 21
CH–1011 Lausanne (Switzerland)
Tel. +41 21 314 0596, Fax +41 21 314 0597, E-Mail Francois.Pralong@chuv.ch

Quinton R (ed): Kallmann Syndrome and Hypogonadotropic Hypogonadism.
Front Horm Res. Basel, Karger, 2010, vol 39, pp 13–24

Role of Kisspeptin/GPR54 System in Human Reproductive Axis

Leticia F.G. Silveira · Milena G. Teles · Ericka B. Trarbach · Ana Claudia Latronico

Unidade de Endocrinologia do Desenvolvimento, Laboratorio de Hormonios e Genetica Molecular – LIM 42, Hospital das Clinicas, Universidade de Sao Paulo, Sao Paulo, Brasil

Abstract

The kisspeptin-GPR54 signaling complex is a key gatekeeper of human sexual maturation. Kisspeptins, encoded by the *KISS1* gene, constitute a powerful stimulus for gonadotropin-releasing hormone-induced gonadotropin secretion. In addition, the *KISS1* gene is a target for regulation by gonadal steroids in both sexes. The increase in hypothalamic kisspeptin expression at puberty is believed to contribute to maturation of the reproductive axis. Homozygous or compound heterozygous loss-of-function mutations in the *GPR54* gene have been identified in familial and sporadic patients with isolated hypogonadotropic hypogonadism without olfactory abnormalities. In addition, mice with targeted deletions of *Kiss1* or *Gpr54* have a similar failure of sexual maturation. Study of these mutations provides an important contribution in the understanding of the role of the kisspeptin/GPR54 system in the control of human puberty development and reproductive function.

The episodic secretion of gonadotropin-releasing hormone (GnRH) from the hypothalamus is the first requirement for the initiation and maintenance of normal reproductive function. In humans, the hypothalamic-pituitary-gonadal axis is fully active in the neonatal life, followed by a period of quiescence during childhood and reactivation in the beginning of puberty. The resurgence of pulsatile GnRH is under the control of a complex network of regulatory signals [1].

Congenital isolated hypogonadotropic hypogonadism (IHH) is defined by partial or complete lack of pubertal development, secondary to deficient GnRH-induced gonadotropin secretion. It is characterized by low levels of sex steroids in the presence of low or inappropriately normal luteinizing hormone (LH) and follicle-stimulating hormone (FSH) serum levels, with no anatomical lesion in the hypothalamo-pituitary tract and no other associated pituitary hormone deficiency [2]. When associated with anosmia, it characterizes Kallmann syndrome [3]. IHH is a rare and genetically heterogeneous condition, which can be sporadic or inherited as an X-linked autosomal recessive or autosomal dominant trait. The diagnosis is typically made in the second or third decade of life, when affected individuals present with delayed pubertal development, primary amenorrhea or infertility [2]. In some cases, the diagnosis may be suspected before puberty, in the presence of microphallus and cryptorchidism, especially in the context of a positive family history [3].

A number of genes involved in different stages of function and development of the hypothalamic-pituitary-gonadal axis have been described. Genes classically implicated in IHH pathogenesis include *KAL1*, associated with X-linked Kallmann syndrome and GnRH receptor *(GnRHR)* associated with normosmic IHH [2]. In recent years, defects in the fibroblast growth factor receptor-1 *(FGFR1)*, fibroblast growth factor-8 *(FGF8)*, prokineticin *(PROK2)* and prokineticin receptor-2 *(PROKR2)* have been identified in cases of Kallmann syndrome and normosmic IHH, suggesting that the same defect can lead to a variable phenotypic spectrum [4–9]. (For an exhaustive list of IHH-related genes, see Pitteloud et al., this volume, pp. 142–153.) Nevertheless, the molecular pathogenesis of the majority of IHH cases remains undefined and the search for new candidate genes is still ongoing.

In the last few years, the interaction between kisspeptins and their receptor (GPR54) has been recognized as a key stimulatory factor for GnRH secretion and is now strongly implicated in the regulation of puberty onset [10–14]. The first evidence that pubertal development was related to the kisspeptin/GPR54 complex appeared in 2003, when loss-of-function mutations of the *GPR54* gene were identified in individuals with normosmic IHH, thereby establishing inactivation of the receptor GPR54 as a new and unsuspected cause of IHH [15, 16]. In this chapter, we review the role of the kisspeptin/GPR54 system in the regulation of reproductive function and consider the implication of GPR54 mutations for human pubertal development.

GPR54 and Kisspeptin

The *Gpr54* gene was cloned in 1999 in the rat as an orphan G-protein-coupled receptor, followed by the identification of its human ortholog [17–19]. The human *GPR54* gene is located at chromosome 19p13.3 and encodes a 398-amino acid heptahelical G-protein-coupled receptor with 40% homology to the galanin receptor family, although galanin itself does not bind to GPR54 [18]. It is expressed mainly in the placenta, hypothalamus, pituitary and pancreas [17, 19, 20].

The isolation from the placenta of peptides with high affinity and agonist activity for the GPR54 receptor led to the description of its endogenous ligands, such that GPR54 was no longer an 'orphan' [17, 19, 20]. These peptides, generically known as kisspeptins, are derived from a precursor peptide encoded by the *KISS1* gene [18, 19]. *KISS1* was originally isolated in a malignant melanoma cell line as a metastasis suppressor gene and mapped to the long arm of chromosome 1 (1q32) [21, 22].

Kisspeptin/GPR54 Signaling Pathway

Binding of kisspeptins to GPR54 results in coupling to the Gαq/11 pathway, with activation of phospholipase C, subsequent phosphatidylinositol biphosphate hydrolysis and accumulation of inositol triphosphate in the cells, leading to intracellular calcium mobilization and protein-kinase C activation and arachidonic acid release [17, 19, 20, 23]. However, kisspeptin action in GnRH neurons also requires the activation of additional signaling mechanisms involving the family of the mitogen-activated protein kinases (MAPKs) [20, 23]. Kisspeptins induce strong sustained stimulation of phosphorylation of the MAPK extracellular signal regulated kinases, ERK1 and ERK2, and a weak stimulation of p38 MAPK phosphorylation [20, 23]. Castellano et al. [24] showed that blocking of the MAPK pathway abolished the kisspeptin-induced GnRH secretion in hypothalamic fragments ex vivo. Nevertheless, the specific pattern of kinases activated by GPR54 stimulation seems to be dependent on the cellular context studied [23].

Animal Studies

The finding that GPR54 inactivation causes IHH in humans motivated a series of pharmacological and physiological studies, which confirmed the crucial role of the kisspeptin/GPR54 system in the hypothalamic-pituitary-gonadal axis activation. The kisspeptins are potent stimulators of GnRH-dependent LH secretion. In mice, intracerebroventricular (i.c.v.) administration of doses as low as 1 fmol of kisspeptin elicited a robust LH and FSH secretion 30 min after the injection [25]. Several administration routes of kisspeptins (i.c.v., subcutaneous, intraperitoneal and intravenous) resulted in similar effects in different mammalian species, including mice, rats, sheep and both human and nonhuman primates [12]. Pretreatment with a GnRH antagonist blocked the kisspeptin-induced LH boost, confirming that the capacity of kisspeptin to stimulate gonadotropin release is dependent on GnRH secretion [25]. In addition, administration of kisspeptin to immature animals was able to induce precocious pubertal development [26, 27]. Intermittent i.c.v. kisspeptin administration to immature female rats for 7 days has been shown to induce precocious activation of the gonadotropic axis, advanced vaginal opening, uterine enlargement, and increased serum levels of LH and estradiol [26].

Likewise, in agonadal juvenile male rhesus monkeys, in which pituitary responsiveness to GnRH had been increased by a priming infusion of exogenous GnRH, intravenous infusions of human kisspeptin-10 every hour, for 48 h, elicited a sustained train of endogenous hypothalamic GnRH discharges, as reflected by the pulsatile pattern of circulating LH concentrations [28]. However, continuous infusion of kisspeptin decreases LH levels in agonadal juvenile male monkeys, suggesting that kisspeptin secretion is probably pulsatile, and the continuous stimulation may induce to desensitization of the receptor – an effect that exactly mirrors that of GnRH on its receptor [29]. Hence the intriguing hypothesis that the pulsatility of GnRH secretion might (at least in part) be entrained through pulsatility of kisspeptin secretion.

Expression Studies

Kisspeptin and GPR54 are widely expressed in human tissues [17, 19, 20]. It has been demonstrated by RT-PCR that *KISS1* mRNA is expressed mainly in the placenta, but also in the brain, including the hypothalamus, basal ganglia, pituitary, and peripheral organs, such as pancreas, testis and, at lower levels, also in the liver and small intestine [17, 19, 20]. *GPR54* transcripts were particularly abundant in placenta, brain, pituitary, spinal cord, and pancreas, whereas lower levels were detected in other tissues, including lymphocytes, spleen, testis and adipose tissue [17, 19, 20].

In situ hybridization study of mouse and rat brains showed that expression of *Kiss1* was highest in the arcuate (ARC) and anteroventral periventricular (AVPV) nuclei, both known to send projections to the medial preoptic area, where there is an abundance of GnRH cell bodies [30]. Moreover, it was demonstrated that GnRH neurons coexpress *Gpr54* transcripts [30]. Hypothalamic *Kiss1* and *Gpr54* mRNA expression increases progressively across the pubertal development, reaching maximum levels at the beginning of puberty in rodents and primates [11, 27]. In male and female rodents, hypothalamic *Kiss1* mRNA expression increased dramatically after bilateral gonadectomy in adult animals and returned to the anterior levels after sexual steroid replacement as demonstrated by immunohistochemistry and in situ hybridization, suggesting an inhibitory effect for the sex steroids [11]. In the AVPV, however, *Kiss1* expression was decreased after gonadectomy and increased after sex steroid replacement in a positive feedback pattern [30, 31]. Moreover, whereas the overall distribution of kisspeptin immunoreactivity was very similar between males and females, the number of cell bodies expressing kisspeptin in the AVPV is over 10-fold higher in the female [32].

The AVPV is one of the only sexually dimorphic areas in the rodent brain that is larger in the female than the male [30]. Virtually all kisspeptin neurons in the ARC and the AVPV were shown to coexpress the estrogen receptor-α (ER-α), whereas only 25–30% of these neurons express the ER-β. Furthermore, ER-β knockout ovariectomized female mice respond to estradiol administration in the same way as the wild-type animals, showing that the estradiol effects are mediated by the ER-α. In males, testosterone effects are mediated by the androgen receptor as well as the ER-α, after testosterone aromatization in estradiol in the ARC. However, in the AVPV, testosterone-induced *Kiss1* transcription seems to be mediated exclusively via ER-α. The ARC is known to control the negative feedback regulation of GnRH and gonadotropin secretion, whereas the estrogen-induced kisspeptin increase in the AVPV seems to be involved in the positive feedback regulation which leads to the preovulatory LH surge in females [30, 33].

In addition to these two hypothalamic nuclei, it was recently demonstrated by immunohistochemistry that kisspeptin and GPR54 are coexpressed by pituitary gonadotrophs, suggesting the possibility of an autocrine or paracrine action of kisspeptin in the pituitary [34]. However, in vitro studies assessing the direct stimulatory effects of kisspeptins on gonadotropin secretion in the pituitary have given conflicting results [35, 36], though Gutierrez-Pascual et al. [37] demonstrated a kisspeptin-10-induced rise in free cytosolic calcium concentration in approximately 10% of male rat pituitary cells, including somatotrophs as well as gonadotrophs.

Gpr54 and *Kiss1* Knockout Mice

Gpr54 and *Kiss1* knockout mice have been generated by different groups of researchers [16, 38–41]. The phenotype of these animals is broadly similar, with slight variations attributable to the type of mutation carried by each line [41]. Both *Gpr54–/–* and *Kiss1–/–* mice fail to undergo pubertal maturation and show poor gonadal development, hypogonadotropic hypogonadism and infertility. Spermatogenesis and ovulation are severely impaired and mutant females do not exhibit estrous cycling. No alterations have been described in organs or systems unrelated to reproduction. The phenotype of *Kiss1–/–* mice does vary, though, from complete IHH similar to *Gpr54–/–* to a less severe phenotype with higher gonadal weight and, in the female animals, more vaginal opening [40]. It is not clear why some *Kiss1–/–* mice have a less marked phenotype than the receptor knockout. One explanation that has been postulated is the ability of another ligand apart from kisspeptin to weakly stimulate GPR54 [40].

The gonads and the anterior pituitary retain functional responses to exogenous GnRH stimulation, consistent with the primary defect being a failure to secrete GnRH from the hypothalamus [41]. However, ex vivo histological examination reveals a normal number of hypothalamic GnRH neurons, of normal morphology, normal intracellular GnRH content and intact axonal projections to the median eminence [16, 39–41]. Thus, unlike the human *KAL1* model of IHH, GnRH neuron migration occurs normally in these mouse models.

When injected with kisspeptin, *Gpr54–/–* mice fail to increase gonadotropins, whereas *Kiss1–/–* and wild-type mice respond with increased gonadotropin secretion, suggesting that kisspeptins act directly and uniquely through GPR54 signaling to stimulate gonadotropin release [40]. In addition, following ovariectomy, *Gpr54–/–* do not respond with a compensatory rise in LH [41].

Taken together, these above observations suggest that the primary defect in these animals is a failure to secrete GnRH from the hypothalamus, evidencing the importance of kisspeptin-mediated GPR54 signaling in GnRH secretion. These two molecules thus constitute an authentic receptor/ligand pair with no obvious redundancy or overlap with other signaling pathways [41].

GPR54-Inactivating Mutations in Humans

GPR54-inactivating mutations were first described in patients with normosmic IHH, almost simultaneously by two independent groups [15, 16]. Both groups identified a new candidate region in the short arm of chromosome 19 using genome-wide scan on large consanguineous IHH families [15, 16]. In 2003, de Roux et al. [15] reported a family with 5 affected siblings with partial normosmic IHH and consanguineous parents. After screening several candidate genes, a homozygous 155 deletion spanning intron 4 and exon 5 of *GPR54* was identified in all affected family members. This deletion removed the intron 4 splicing site, resulting in a truncated protein of 247 amino acids. By contrast, the nonaffected members were either heterozygous or homozygous for the wild-type sequence [15].

In the same year, Seminara et al. [16] studied a large consanguineous Saudi Arabian family with 6 members affected with normosmic IHH (4 males and 2 females). All affected members harbored a homozygous missense mutation in exon 3 of the *GPR54* gene. A change of thymine by a cytosine at position 443 resulted in the substitution of leucine by a serine at position 148 (p.L148S) in the second intracellular loop of the protein. Affected individuals had partial response to acute GnRH stimulation test, and 4 of them underwent fertility therapy with either exogenous gonadotropins or pulsatile GnRH, with successful responses in all cases. In the same study, a compound heterozygous mutation [p.(R331X) + (X399R)] was identified in an African-American patient with sporadic normosmic IHH. The hormonal evaluation of this patient showed low levels of basal LH in a sampling period of 24 h, although low-amplitude pulses of LH were detected, suggesting reduced secretion of GnRH. After four doses of intravenous GnRH, the dose-response curve was leftward shifted when compared to other patients with IHH without GPR54 mutations, suggesting an increased sensibility to exogenous GnRH [16].

Functional studies were performed using COS-7 cells transfected with three different mutant GPR54 receptors (p.L148S, p.R331X and p.X399R). The in vitro analysis demonstrated a reduction in the signaling capacity after kisspeptin-10 stimulation in cells containing the mutant receptors, evidenced by reduced intracellular accumulation of inositol phosphate [16]. These findings demonstrated for the first time that

Table 1. GPR54 inactivating mutations in IHH

Case	Mutation (cDNA)	Mutation (protein)	Patient's status	Familial/ sporadic	Affected members	References
1	IVS4-13-42del155	truncated protein	homozygous	familial	4M + 1F	[15]
2	c.443T>C	p.L148S	homozygous	familial	4M + 2F	[16]
3	c.991C>T/ c.1195T>A	p.R331X/ p.X399R	compound heterozygous	sporadic	M	[16]
4	c.667T>C/ c.891G>T	p.C223R/ p.R297L	compound heterozygous	sporadic	M	[42]
5	c.1101_1002insC	frameshift	homozygous	sporadic	M	[44]
6	c.305T>C	p.L102P	homozygous	familial	1M + 2F	[43]
7	c.305T>C	p.L102P	homozygous	familial	2M + 2F	[43]
8	IVS2-4-2delGCinsACCGGCT	truncated protein	homozygous	familial	2M	[45]

M = Male; F = female.

inactivating mutations of GPR54 receptor could be a cause of normosmic IHH in humans [15, 16].

Since then, other homozygous or compound heterozygous inactivating mutations have been identified in the GPR54 gene in patients with IHH, characterizing the autosomal recessive pattern of this condition [15, 16, 42–45] (table 1; fig. 1). In 2005, Semple et al. [42] screened 30 patients with IHH or delayed puberty for mutations in the *GPR54* and *KISS1* genes. One patient with IHH detected at birth due to bilateral cryptorchidism and micropenis carried compound heterozygous GPR54 mutations, characterized by the change of a cysteine for arginine at position 223 in the fifth transmembrane helix, and the substitution of a leucine by arginine [p.(C223R) + (R297L)] in the third extracellular loop of the receptor. In vitro studies of the p.C223R mutation showed a decrease of 80% of the signaling capacity. However, functional studies of the p.R297L GPR54 mutant showed only a mild impairment of its function [42]. Regarding the *KISS1* gene, only polymorphisms were identified in this study [42].

In the same year, Lanfranco et al. [44] described a homozygous *GPR54* mutation, c.1001_1002insC, in one patient with sporadic IHH and consanguineous parents of German descent. This insertion was located at the seventh transmembrane helix of the receptor, resulting in a frameshift in the open reading frame and elongation of 43 amino acids with an increased number of proline residues in the intracellular receptor domain [44]. This patient presented with delayed puberty and bilateral undescended

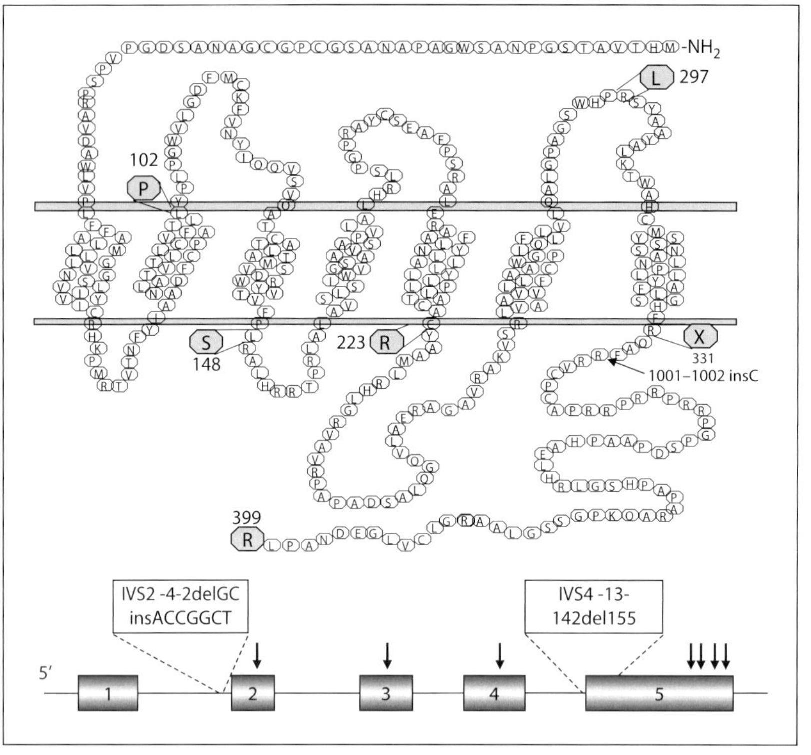

Fig. 1. Schematic representation of GPR54 receptor (top) and *GPR54* gene (bottom) showing the location of all published inactivating mutations causing IHH.

testes. Hormonal evaluation showed moderately low LH (1.1 IU/l) and FSH (2.2 IU/l) levels along with reduced testosterone (3.4 nM), but normal gonadotropin response to acute GnRH administration. At the age of 31, pulsatile GnRH therapy (5 mg/120 min s.c.) was started and after 2 years of treatment he achieved sperm maturation sufficient to induce pregnancy with assisted fertilization [44].

In 2006, Tenenbaum-Rakover et al. [43] described a novel *GPR54* missense mutation in the homozygous state in two unrelated, consanguineous Arab families. A substitution of a cytosine for thymidine in the position 305, in the exon 2, resulted in a proline substitution for leucine at position 102 (p.L102P). Functional studies showed a complete reduction of inositol generation after kisspeptin-10 stimulation [43]. Affected patients with the p.L102P mutation showed variable responses to GnRH acute stimulation test. A 9-year follow-up of one of the probands revealed progressive changes in pituitary response. The LH and FSH levels after GnRH stimulus progressively increased across the follow-up from prepubertal to almost pubertal levels around 21 years of age. This finding suggested that the p.L102P inactivating mutation leads to a more quantitative than qualitative defect of gonadotropic axis activation [43].

A novel homozygous *GPR54* gene mutation in 2 Brazilian siblings with normosmic IHH was recently identified by our group [45]. This insertion/deletion mutation was characterized by the deletion of three nucleotides (GCA) at positions −2 to −4, and the insertion of seven nucleotides (ACCGGCT) within the 3′ splice acceptor site of intron 2. Computational splice site analysis suggests that this change is predicted to generate a truncated protein. This variant was absent in 240 control alleles. The 2 affected brothers presented with micropenis and had no clinical evidence of pubertal development at age 14 and 20 years, respectively. Both exhibited low basal gonadotropins with prepubertal testosterone levels. Their mother carried the same mutation in the heterozygous state and had normal pubertal development [43].

In summary, nine different inactivating mutations have been identified in the *GPR54* gene in patients with IHH so far. The studies above demonstrated that *GPR54* mutations are a rare cause of IHH, being responsible for less than 5% of all reported IHH cases, although this prevalence is higher in familial cases. GPR54 abnormalities were identified in 3 out of 180 sporadic cases (1.6%) and 5 of 24 familial cases (20.8%) [15, 16, 42–45]. Affected patients presented with impaired pubertal development with no other associated condition. Micropenis and cryptorchidism were described in 3 and 2 cases, respectively, suggesting a role for kisspeptin in the gonadotropin-induced androgen secretion in the last trimester of gestation [15, 16, 42–45]. The gonadotropin secretion in response to acute GnRH test was variable from blunted to normal [16, 43, 44]. Notably, some of the patients with GPR54 mutations were successfully treated with pulsatile GnRH therapy and achieved sperm maturation and fertility, confirming data from animal models that the kisspeptin-GPR54 system operates hierarchically above the level of GnRH-GnRHR interaction [16, 41, 43, 44].

Perspectives

In the last few years, kisspeptin and its receptor GPR54 were revealed as the key regulators of puberty onset. Although inactivating mutations in GPR54 are a rare cause of IHH, the study of these mutations is critical to the understanding of the gene function and the role of the kisspeptin/GPR54 system in the control of human puberty development and reproductive function.

Given the undisputed importance of the kisspeptin/GPR54 complex for pubertal development, the involvement of these genes in the pathogenesis of other central pubertal disorders, including central (gonadotropin-dependent) precocious puberty might also be expected. Significantly, a nonconstitutively activating autosomal dominant point mutation of GPR54 (ARG386Pro) has recently been reported as a cause of idiopathic central precocious puberty in an 8-year-old girl [46]. When the mutant receptor was transfected into COS-7 cells, the phenotype was of prolonged receptor activation, evidenced by the protracted elevation of inositol phosphate [46].

References

1 Palmert MR, Boepple PA: Variation in the timing of puberty: clinical spectrum and genetic investigation. J Clin Endocrinol Metab 2001;86:2364–2368.

2 Seminara SB, Oliveira LM, Beranova M, Hayes FJ, Crowley WF Jr: Genetics of hypogonadotrophic hypogonadism. J Endocrinol Invest 2000;23:560–565.

3 Quinton R, Duke VM, Robertson A, Kirk JM, Matfin G, de Zoysa PA, Azcona C, MacColl GS, Jacobs HS, Conway GS, Besser M, Stanhope RG, Bouloux P-MG: Idiopathic gonadotropin deficiency: genetic questions addressed through phenotypic characterization. Clin Endocrinol (Oxf) 2001; 55:163–174.

4 Falardeau J, Chung WC, Beenken A, Raivio T, Plummer L, Sidis Y, Jacobson-Dickman EE, Eliseenkova AV, Ma J, Dwyer AA, Quinton R, Na S, Hall JE, Huot C, Alois N, Pearce SH, Cole LW, Hughes VA, Mohammadi M, Tsai PS, Pitteloud N: Decreased FGF8 signalling causes deficiency of gonadotropin-releasing hormone in humans and mice. J Clin Invest 2008;118:2822–2231.

5 Trarbach EB, Silveira LG, Latronico AC: Genetic insights into human isolated gonadotropin deficiency. Pituitary 2007;10:381–391.

6 Cole LW, Sidis Y, Zhang C, Quinton R, Plummer L, Pignatelli D, Hughes VA, Dwyer AA, Raivio T, Hayes FJ, Seminara SB, Huot C, Alos N, Speiser P, Takeshita A, Van Vliet G, Pearce SH, Crowley WF Jr, Zhou QY, Pitteloud N: Mutations in prokineticin 2 (PROK2) and PROK2 receptor (PROKR2) in human gonadotropin-releasing hormone deficiency: molecular genetics and clinical spectrum. J Clin Endocrinol Metab 2008;93:3551–3559.

7 Abreu AP, Trarbach EB, de Castro M, Frade Costa EM, Versiani B, Baptista MT, Garmes HM, Mendonca BB, Latronico AC: Loss-of-function mutations in the genes encoding prokineticin-2 or prokineticin receptor-2 cause autosomal recessive Kallmann syndrome. J Clin Endocrinol Metab 2008; 93:4113–4118.

8 Raivio T, Sidis Y, Plummer L, Chen H, Ma J, Mukherjee A, Jacobson-Dickman E, Quinton R, Van Vliet G, Lavoie H, Hughes VA, Dwyer AA, Hayes FJ, Xu S, Sparks S, Kaiser UB, Mohammadi M, Pitteloud N: Impaired fibroblast growth factor receptor 1 signaling as a cause of normosmic idiopathic hypogonadotropic hypogonadism. J Clin Endocrinol Metab 2009;94:4380–4390.

9 Trarbach EB, Teles MG, Costa EM, Abreu AP, Garmes HM, Guerra G Jr, et al: Screening of autosomal gene deletions in patients with hypogonadotropic hypogonadism using multiplex ligation-dependent probe amplification: detection of a hemizygosis for the fibroblast growth factor receptor 1. Clin Endocrinol (Oxf) 2009, Epub ahead of print.

10 Han SK, Gottsch ML, Lee KJ, Popa SM, Smith JT, Jakawich SK, Clifton DK, Steiner RA, Herbison AE: Activation of gonadotropin-releasing hormone neurons by kisspeptin as a neuroendocrine switch for the onset of puberty. J Neurosci 2005;25:11349–11356.

11 Navarro VM, Castellano JM, Fernández-Fernández R, Barreiro ML, Roa J, Sanchez-Criado JE, Aguilar E, Dieguez C, Pinilla L, Tena-Sempere M: Developmental and hormonally regulated messenger ribonucleic acid expression of KiSS-1 and its putative receptor, GPR54, in rat hypothalamus and potent luteinizing hormone-releasing activity of KiSS-1 peptide. Endocrinology 2004;145:4565–4574.

12 Navarro VM, Castellano JM, Garcia-Galiano D, Tena-Sempere M: Neuroendocrine factors in the initiation of puberty: the emergent role of kisspeptin. Rev Endocr Metab Disord 2007;8:11–20.

13 Seminara SB: Mechanisms of disease: the first kiss – a crucial role for kisspeptin-1 and its receptor, G-protein-coupled receptor 54, in puberty and reproduction. Nat Clin Pract Endocrinol Metab 2006;2:328–234.

14 Messager S, Chatzidaki EE, Ma D, Hendrick AG, Zahn D, Dixon J, Thresher RR, Malinge I, Lomet D, Carlton MB, Colledge WH, Caraty A, Aparicio SA: Kisspeptin directly stimulates gonadotropin-releasing hormone release via G protein-coupled receptor 54. Proc Natl Acad Sci USA 2005;102;1761–1766.

15 de Roux N, Genin E, Carel JC, Matsuda F, Chaussain JL, Milgrom E: Hypogonadotrophic hypogonadism due to loss of function of the KiSS1-derived peptide receptor GPR54. Proc Natl Acad Sci USA 2003;100: 10972–10976.

16 Seminara SB, Messager S, Chatzidaki EE, Thresher RR, Acierno JS Jr, Shagoury JK, Bo-Abbas Y, Kuohung W, Schwinof KM, Hendrick AG, Zahn D, Dixon J, Kaiser UB, Slaugenhaupt SA, Gusella JF, O'Rahilly S, Carlton MB, Crowley WF Jr, Aparicio SA, Colledge WH: The GPR54 gene as a regulator of puberty. N Engl J Med 2003;349:1614–1627.

17 Ohtaki T, Shintani Y, Honda S, Matsumoto H, Hori A, Kanehashi K, Terao Y, Kumano S, Takatsu Y, Masuda Y, Ishibashi Y, Watanabe T, Asada M, Yamada T, Suenaga M, Kitada C, Usuki S, Kurokawa T, Onda H, Nishimura O, Fujino M: Metastasis suppressor gene KiSS-1 encodes peptide ligand of a G-protein-coupled receptor. Nature 2001;411:613–617.

18 Lee DK, Nguyen T, O'Neill GP, Cheng R, Liu Y, Howard AD, Coulombe N, Tan CP, Tang-Nguyen AT, George SR, O'Dowd BF: Discovery of a receptor related to the galanin receptors. FEBS Lett 1999; 446:103–107.

19 Muir AI, Chamberlain L, Elshourbagy NA, Michalovich D, Moore DJ, Calamari A, Szekeres PG, Sarau HM, Chambers JK, Murdock P, Steplewski K, Shabon U, Miller JE, Middleton SE, Darker JG, Larminie CG, Wilson S, Bergsma DJ, Emson P, Faull R, Philpott KL, Harrison DC: AXOR12, a novel human G protein-coupled receptor, activated by the peptide KiSS-1. J Biol Chem 2001;276:28969–28975.

20 Kotani M, Detheux M, Vandenbogaerde A, Communi D, Vanderwinden JM, Le Poul E, Brézillon S, Tyldesley R, Suarez-Huerta N, Vandeput F, Blanpain C, Schiffmann SN, Vassart G, Parmentier M: The metastasis suppressor gene KiSS-1 encodes kisspeptins, the natural ligands of the orphan G protein-coupled receptor GPR54. J Biol Chem 2001; 276:34631–34636.

21 Lee JH, Miele ME, Hicks DJ, Phillips KK, Trent JM, Weissman BE, Welch DR: KiSS-1, a novel human malignant melanoma metastasis-suppressor gene. J Natl Cancer Inst 1996;88:1731–1737.

22 West A, Vojta PJ, Welch DR, Weissman BE: Chromosome localization and genomic structure of the KiSS-1 metastasis suppressor gene (KISS1). Genomics 1998;54:145–148.

23 Castano JP, Martinez-Fuentes AJ, Gutierrez-Pascual E, Vaudry H, Tena-Sempere M, Malagon MM: Intracellular signalling pathways activated by kisspeptins through GPR54: Do multiple signals underlie function diversity? Peptides 2008;30:10–15.

24 Castellano JM, Navarro VM, Fernández-Fernández R, Castaño JP, Malagón MM, Aguilar E, Dieguez C, Magni P, Pinilla L, Tena-Sempere M: Ontogeny and mechanisms of action for the stimulatory effect of kisspeptin on gonadotropin-releasing hormone system of the rat. Mol Cell Endocrinol 2006;257–258: 75–83.

25 Gottsch ML, Cunningham MJ, Smith JT, Popa SM, Acohido BV, Crowley WF, Seminara SB, Clifton DK, Steiner RA: A role for kisspeptins in the regulation of gonadotropin secretion in the mouse. Endocrinology 2004;145:4073–4077.

26 Navarro VM, Fernández-Fernández R, Castellano JM, Roa J, Mayen A, Barreiro ML, Gaytan F, Aguilar E, Pinilla L, Dieguez C, Tena-Sempere M: Advanced vaginal opening and precocious activation of the reproductive axis by KiSS-1 peptide, the endogenous ligand of GPR54. J Physiol 2004;561:379–386.

27 Shahab M, Mastronardi C, Seminara SB, Crowley WF, Ojeda SR, Plant TM: Increased hypothalamic GPR54 signalling: a potential mechanism for initiation of puberty in primates. Proc Natl Acad Sci USA 2005;102:2129–2134.

28 Plant TM, Ramaswamy S, Dipietro MJ: Repetitive activation of hypothalamic G protein-coupled receptor 54 with intravenous pulses of kisspeptin in the juvenile monkey *(Macaca mulatta)* elicits a sustained train of gonadotropin-releasing hormone discharges. Endocrinology 2006;147:1007–1013.

29 Seminara SB, Dipietro MJ, Ramaswamy S, Crowley WF Jr, Plant TM: Continuous human metastin 45–54 infusion desensitizes G protein-coupled receptor 54-induced gonadotropin-releasing hormone release monitored indirectly in the juvenile male Rhesus monkey *(Macaca mulatta)*: a finding with therapeutic implications. Endocrinology 2006; 147:2122–2126.

30 Smith JT, Clarke IJ: Kisspeptin expression in the brain: catalyst for the initiation of puberty. Rev Endocr Metab Disord 2007;8:1–9.

31 Smith JT, Cunningham MJ, Rissman EF, Clifton DK, Steiner RA: Regulation of Kiss1 gene expression in the brain of the female mouse. Endocrinology 2005;146:3686–3692.

32 Clarkson J, Herbison AE: Postnatal development of kisspeptin neurons in mouse hypothalamus; sexual dimorphism and projections to gonadotropin-releasing hormone neurons. Endocrinology 2006; 147:5817–5825.

33 Gottsch ML, Clifton DK, Steiner RA: Kisspepeptin GPR54 signalling in the neuroendocrine reproductive axis. Mol Cell Endocrinol 2006;254–255:91–96.

34 Richard N, Galmiche G, Corvaisier S, Caraty A, Kottler ML: KiSS-1 and GPR54 genes are co-expressed in rat gonadotrophs and differentially regulated in vivo by oestradiol and gonadotropin-releasing hormone. J Neuroendocrinol 2008;20:381–393.

35 Richard N, Corvaisier S, Camacho E, Kottler ML: KiSS-1 and GPR54 at the pituitary level: overview and recent insights. Peptides 2008;30:123–139.

36 Ramaswamy S, Gibbs RB, Plant TM: Studies of the localisation of kisspeptin within the pituitary of the rhesus monkey *(Macaca mulatta)* and the effect of kisspeptin on the release of non-gonadotropic pituitary hormones. J Neuroendocrinol 2009;21:795–804.

37 Gutierrez-Pascual E, Martinez-Fuentes AJ, Pinilla L, Tena-Sempere M, Malagon MM, Castano JP: Direct pituitary effects of kisspeptin: activation of gonadotrophs and somatotrophs and stimulation of luteinising hormone and growth hormone secretion. J Neuroendocrinol 2007;19:521–530.
38 Funes S, Hedrick JA, Vassileva G, Markowitz L, Abbondanzo S, Golovko A, Yang S, Monsma FJ, Gustafson EL: The KiSS-1 receptor GPR54 is essential for the development of the murine reproductive system. Biochem Biophys Res Commun 2003;312: 1357–1363.
39 d'Anglemont de Tassigny X, Fagg LA, Dixon JP, Day K, Leitch HG, Hendrick AG, Zahn D, Franceschini I, Caraty A, Carlton MB, Aparicio SA, Colledge WH: Hypogonadotrophic hypogonadism in mice lacking a functional Kiss1 gene. Proc Natl Acad Sci USA 2007;104:10714–10719.
40 Lapatto R, Pallais JC, Zhang D, Chan YM, Mahan A, Cerrato F, Le WW, Hoffman GE, Seminara SB: Kiss1–/– mice exhibit more variable hypogonadism than Gpr54–/– mice. Endocrinology 2007;148:4927–4936.
41 Colledge WH: Transgenic mouse models to study Gpr54/kisspeptin physiology. Peptides 2009;30:34–41.
42 Semple RK, Achermann JC, Ellery J, Farooqi IS, Karet FE, Stanhope RG, O'Rahilly S, Aparicio SA: Two novel missense mutations in g protein-coupled receptor 54 in a patient with hypogonadotrophic hypogonadism. J Clin Endocrinol Metab 2005;90: 1849–1855.
43 Tenenbaum-Rakover Y, Commenges-Ducos M, Iovane A, Aumas C, Admoni O, de Roux N: Neuroendocrine phenotype analysis in five patients with isolated hypogonadotrophic hypogonadism due to a L102P inactivating mutation of GPR54. J Clin Endocrinol Metab 2007;92:1137–1144.
44 Lanfranco F, Gromoll J, von Eckardstein S, Herding EM, Nieschlag E, Simoni M: Role of sequence variations of the GnRH receptor and G protein-coupled receptor 54 gene in male idiopathic hypogonadotrophic hypogonadism. Eur J Endocrinol 2005;153:845–852.
45 Teles MG, Trarbach EB, Guerra G, Costa EMF, Baptista MT, Castro M, Mendonca BB, Kaiser UB, Latronico AC: A novel splice site mutation in GPR54 in two siblings with normosmic isolated hypogonadotrophic hypogonadism. Endocr Soc Annu Meet 2007, Toronto, Canada.
46 Teles MG, Bianco SD, Brito VN, Trarbach EB, Kuohung W, Xu S, Seminara SB, Mendonca BB, Kaiser UB, Latronico AC: A GPR54-activating mutation in a patient with central precocious puberty. N Engl J Med 2008;358:709–715.

Leticia F.G. Silveira, MD
Disciplina de Endocrinologia e Metabologia
Hospital das Clinicas, Faculdade de Medicina da Universidade de Sao Paulo
Av. Dr. Eneas de Carvalho Aguiar, 155, 2° andar, Bloco 6
São Paulo, SP 05403–900 (Brasil)
Tel. +55 11 30697512, Fax +55 11 30697519, E-Mail leticia_gontijo@yahoo.com.br

Quinton R (ed): Kallmann Syndrome and Hypogonadotropic Hypogonadism.
Front Horm Res. Basel, Karger, 2010, vol 39, pp 25–36

Biology of Kisspeptins

Saira Hameed · Waljit S. Dhillo

Section of Investigative Medicine, Faculty of Medicine, Imperial College London, Hammersmith Hospital, London, UK

Abstract

In recent years, a substantial body of evidence has accumulated suggesting that the hypothalamic peptide hormone kisspeptin and its cognate receptor, G-protein-coupled receptor 54, play a fundamental role both as gatekeepers for the initiation of puberty and in the regulation of the hypothalamic-pituitary-gonadal axis. This review discusses the physiology of the kisspeptin signalling system and examines how findings from animal and human studies have contributed to our understanding of the pathophysiology of idiopathic hypogonadotropic hypogonadism.

Idiopathic hypogonadotropic hypogonadism (IHH) occurs in the presence of low levels of circulating gonadotropins, which results in impaired gonadal function with reduced levels of sex steroids. Such a state is termed idiopathic when it arises in the absence of a hypothalamic or a pituitary lesion, and with otherwise normal pituitary function. It is sometimes termed normosmic IHH to distinguish it more clearly from Kallmann syndrome, where olfaction is absent or impaired. The novel hypothalamic peptide kisspeptin and its cognate receptor G-protein-coupled receptor 54 (GPR54) are emerging as key players in the regulation of the hypothalamic-pituitary-gonadal (HPG) axis and are providing new insights into the pathophysiology of IHH.

Discovery of Kisspeptin

Kisspeptin is a peptide hormone, so named because it was discovered in Hershey Pennsylvania, where Hershey Kiss™ chocolate is manufactured. Kisspeptin was originally isolated following the observation that the transfer of chromosome 6 into two human melanoma cell lines reduced the metastatic potential of the tumour cells without affecting cellular proliferation or migration [1]. In the search to identify the gene responsible for this observation, a modified subtractive hybridisation technique was employed in order to compare mRNA expression in metastatic and non-metastatic hybrid clones containing the transferred chromosome 6. This led to the discovery of a novel cDNA, *KiSS-1*, present only in the suppressed melanoma cell line [1].

Distribution of *KiSS-1*

Northern blot hybridisation studies have revealed that the expression of peripheral *KiSS-1* mRNA is highest in human placenta [2]. In the periphery, *KiSS-1* gene expression has also been identified in the testis, pancreas, liver and small intestine [2]. In the central nervous system (CNS), in situ hybridisation studies performed on mouse brains have demonstrated significant *KiSS-1* mRNA expression in the hypothalamic arcuate nucleus (ARC), anteroventral periventricular nucleus (AVPV) and periventricular (PeN) nucleus [3], regions of the hypothalamus that are known to be important in the regulation of gonadotropin secretion. Further work has demonstrated kisspeptin protein expression in these same areas [4]. In addition, *KiSS-1* is also expressed in male and female rat gonadotrophs [5]. A study on human brain tissue using quantitative real-time PCR and immunohistochemistry has demonstrated extra-hypothalamic *KiSS-1* expression, particularly within the basal ganglia, although the physiological role of this expression has not been determined [6].

Kisspeptin Structure

The kisspeptins are a family of peptide hormones, which exist in four bioactive forms, kisspeptin-54, -14, -13 and -10, the suffix denoting the number of amino acids [7]. All forms of kisspeptin are produced by the post-translational cleavage of the 145-amino acid, hydrophilic *KiSS-1* gene product. Kisspeptin belongs to the RF family of neuropeptides which all terminate with an arginine and phenylalanine residue at the amino terminus [Arg-Phe-NH2] [8]. The presence of pairs of basic residues within the full-length gene product, flanking the 54-amino acid peptide, has led to the suggestion that kisspeptin 54 may be produced following cleavage by furin or prohormone convertases [7]. The 14-, 13- and 10-amino acid peptides are present within the 54-amino acid peptide and are likely to be produced by proteolytic degradation within the plasma. The relative importance of the C-terminal and the RF-amide moieties has been demonstrated by the efficacy and affinity of the shorter fragments at the GPR54 receptor [7]. In addition, synthetic kisspeptins lacking any one of the 10 residues of the RF-amide sequence are unable to bind and generate a functional receptor response [7]. These findings suggest that this C-terminal portion is essential for receptor binding and activation.

G-Protein-Coupled Receptor 54

Following a PCR search of rat brain cDNA, GPR54 was cloned and identified as having 38% sequence homology with the rat galanin receptor at the amino acid level, although GPR54 does not bind galanin in vitro [9]. GPR54 is a member of the rhodopsin family of G-protein-coupled receptors and was originally part of the orphan receptor family of receptors defined by the absence of an identified endogenous ligand. The discovery that kisspeptin was its cognate ligand was made 2 years after GPR54 was first cloned, following transfection of GPR54 into a reporter cell line and then screening for intracellular calcium mobilisation following exposure to a panel of peptide ligands [8]. This was a somewhat unexpected finding since a feature of receptors that bind the RF-amides is the presence of an extracellular aspartic acid residue within transmembrane domain six that has been postulated to be important for ligand binding [10], but is not found in GPR54.

In the CNS, GPR54 is widely expressed both in cortical and subcortical regions with the highest expression in the amygdala and hypothalamus [9], a pattern of expression that is similar to that of galanin receptors.

GPR54 Is Expressed on Gonadotropin-Releasing Hormone Neurons

Immunohistochemistry studies have demonstrated that within the hypothalamus, GPR54 co-localises with gonadotropin-releasing hormone (GnRH) neuronal cell bodies and dendrites [11]. Light microscopy using the immunoperoxidase technique has shown that GnRH neurons are present in the mediobasal hypothalamus (MBH), in a continuum from the septal-preoptic region anteriorly to the premammillary nucleus posteriorly, with reactive axons present in the median eminence [12]. Electrophysiological studies have demonstrated bursts of electrical activity within the MBH, including the ARC, which can be correlated with the pulsatile release of luteinising hormone (LH) from the anterior pituitary gland [13], and lesions of the ARC abolish neural control of gonadotropin secretion [14].

Kisspeptin Stimulates GnRH and Gonadotropin Release

The intracerebroventricular (ICV) and peripheral administration of kisspeptin to rats leads to a marked rise in plasma LH, follicle-stimulating hormone (FSH) and total testosterone in male rats [15, 16]. Furthermore, the application of kisspeptin-10 to hypothalamic explants leads to GnRH release [16]. Electrophysiological studies have shown that this excitatory effect of kisspeptin on GnRH neurons is due to the closure of membrane-bound potassium channels and the opening of non-selective cation channels [17]. Two hours after ICV administration of kisspeptin-52 to male rats, expression of the immediate early gene *fos*, an established marker of a marker of neuronal activation [18, 19], is markedly increased in GnRH neurons [20]. The application of a synthetic antagonist of GPR54 leads to potent inhibition of GnRH neuronal firing in mouse brain slices, and an attenuated kisspeptin-induced LH response in male rats [21]. Furthermore, when rats are pre-treated with the GnRH antagonist acyline prior to the ICV administration of kisspeptin the expected rise in LH following kisspeptin administration is prevented [20]. Kisspeptin signalling has also been shown to be essential for the LH surge preceding ovulation in a mouse model since exogenous oestrogen induced the LH surge in wild-type ovariectomised mice, but it failed to do so in either GPR54 (GPR54–/–) or *KiSS-1* (*KiSS-1*–/–) knockout mice [22]. In sum, these studies suggest that kisspeptin stimulates GnRH release.

The stimulatory effect of kisspeptin on the HPG axis has also been demonstrated in humans. In a double-blind, placebo-controlled, crossover study, 6 healthy male volunteers received an intravenous infusion of kisspeptin-54 and a control saline infusion [23]. Kisspeptin-54 infusion significantly increased plasma LH, FSH, and testosterone. The subcutaneous (sc) administration of kisspeptin-54 to pre-menopausal female subjects induces a similar rise in plasma LH, and this effect was most marked in the pre-ovulatory phase [24]. In women with hypothalamic amenorrhea, the sc administration of kisspeptin-54 potently increases plasma LH and FSH at the first injection, but this effect is markedly diminished following 14 days of twice daily kisspeptin-54 injection [25].

Kisspeptin Signal Transduction within GnRH Neurons

In vitro work using GPR54 expressed in a reporter cell line has demonstrated that the binding of kisspeptin leads to intracellular calcium mobilisation as detected by the production of β-lactamase following receptor activation [8]. This may be secondary to activation of the inositol phosphate pathway since phosphatidylinositol turnover is increased following GPR54 activation by kisspeptin [7]. Furthermore, application of antagonists of phospholipase C and of inositol triphosphate receptors to GnRH neurons in vitro before exposure of the cells to kisspeptin leads to a significant reduction in the neuronal response to kisspeptin [17].

Kisspeptin Does Not Affect GnRH Neuronal Migration

The consequence of this GnRH neuronal activation by kisspeptin was initially postulated to influence cellular migration. Two strands of evidence seemed to support this hypothesis; the first was the anti-metastatic properties of kisspeptin, which included its in vitro anti-chemotactic properties in CHO cells transfected with GPR54 [2], human breast carcinoma cells [26] and a melanoma cell line [1].

Secondly, some cases of hypogonadotropic hypogonadism are due to the abnormal migration of GnRH neurons during embryological development. This finding is best described in the X-linked recessive form of Kallmann syndrome in which deficiency of the cell adhesion molecule anosmin, the protein product of the *KAL1* gene, results in the abnormal migration of GnRH neurons from the olfactory placode to the hypothalamus [27, 28].

However, further work has shown that kisspeptin is unlikely to play a major role in GnRH neuronal migration. In particular, compelling evidence comes from studies on GPR54–/– [11, 29] and *KiSS-1–/–* [30, 31] knockout mice in which histological examination ex vivo reveals anatomically normal GnRH neurons which have the expected axonal projections to the median eminence and normal amounts of GnRH within the cells [11].

Effect of Kisspeptin on Gonadotrophs

Whether kisspeptin exerts a physiologically relevant stimulatory effect on gonadotropin secretion at the level of the anterior pituitary has been subject to some controversy. Immunocytochemistry studies have demonstrated that both the *GPR54* and *KiSS-1* genes are co-expressed in rat gonadotrophs and that expression of the latter is positively regulated by estradiol [5]. Furthermore, treatment of rat gonadotrophs with kisspeptin-10 leads to a rise in cytosolic free calcium and a dose-related LH secretory response [32].

However, this in vitro kisspeptin-induced rise in gonadotropins following application to pituitary fragments has not been replicated by other investigators [16]. In an in vivo model, the administration of kisspeptin to hypothalamo-pituitary disconnected ewes fails to induce a rise in LH secretion [33]. Furthermore, the prevention of the kisspeptin-induced LH rise in male monkeys [34] following pre-treatment with a GnRH antagonist would imply that the stimulatory effects of kisspeptin on gonadotropin release are through GnRH. In addition, GPR54 knockout mice have functionally intact pituitary gonadotrophs with an appropriate response to administered GnRH [35].

Regulation of Kisspeptin Signalling

Throughout most of the menstrual cycle, oestrogen exerts a negative feedback effect on gonadotropin secretion, but at mid-cycle, the effect of oestrogen on the HPG axis changes to a potent positive feedback effect, leading to a surge in plasma LH and ovulation.

The oestrogen receptor (ER) is an intra-nuclear receptor which exists in two forms, ERα and ERβ. The importance of hypothalamic ERα for gonadal hormone positive feedback on GnRH release is demonstrated in neuron-specific ER mutant mice in which the mid-cycle gonadotropin surge is preserved in the ERβ mutants but absent in the ERα mutant animals [36]. However, GnRH neurons express ERβ but not ERα [37], implying that the positive feedback effect of oestrogen on GnRH secretion may be mediated indirectly by the action of ERα-expressing neurons, which in turn stimulate GnRH neurons. Using a Cre-dependent, GnRH neuron-specific Pseudorabies virus tracing approach, these ERα-expressing neurons have been identified in the PeN, AVPV, median pre-optic nucleus and ARC [36], areas that have been shown to express *KiSS-1* mRNA [3]. Furthermore, dual in situ hybridisation studies have shown that almost all neurons in the ARC and AVPV which express *KiSS-1* also express ERα [38].

In female rats, following oestrogen treatment, there is a significant change in c-*fos* expression in *KiSS-1* mRNA expressing neurons in the AVPV, but not the ARC [39]. Furthermore, AVPV *KiSS-1* expression is reduced after ovariectomy in female mice but increased following oestrogen replacement in the castrate animals [37]. Administration of anti-rat kisspeptin monoclonal antibody into the preoptic area blocks the oestrogen-stimulated LH rise in female rats and the administration of a kisspeptin antagonist blocks the post-castration rise in LH in orchidectomised rats and mice and ovariectomised ewes [21, 39].

In castrated male rats, in situ hybridisation studies have demonstrated significantly higher levels of *KiSS-1* mRNA in the ARC compared with control animals [20]. Conversely, testosterone replacement reduces the expression of kisspeptin in the MBH [40]. *KiSS-1* expression in the ARC is also increased in female mice following ovariectomy, and this is reversed by the administration of estradiol [38]. These findings suggest that *KiSS-1* gene expression in the ARC is negatively regulated and in the AVPV positively regulated by feedback from gonadal hormones (fig. 1).

Continuous Administration of Kisspeptin Leads to Desensitisation to Its Effects

The continuous intravenous infusion of the C-terminal fragment of kisspeptin (112–121) to juvenile male agonadal *Macaca mulatta* monkeys over 4 days, following initial priming with GnRH boluses, leads to the brisk, expected rise in plasma LH [41]. However, this effect is short lived, lasting only 1–2 hours, following which, despite continuous infusion, kisspeptin does not elevate plasma LH levels [41]. At the end of this study, the ability of GnRH boluses to elicit LH pulses demonstrates that the low plasma LH reflects desensitisation of the HPG axis to kisspeptin following its continuous administration, rather than a loss of integral axis integrity. Thus, it seems that, as with the stimulation of gonadotrophs by GnRH [42], for kisspeptin to effectively stimulate gonadotropin release, stimulation of GnRH neurons by kisspeptin needs to be intermittent. The mechanism of this desensitisation has not been elucidated. Likewise, the response to exogenous GnRH administration is preserved in women with

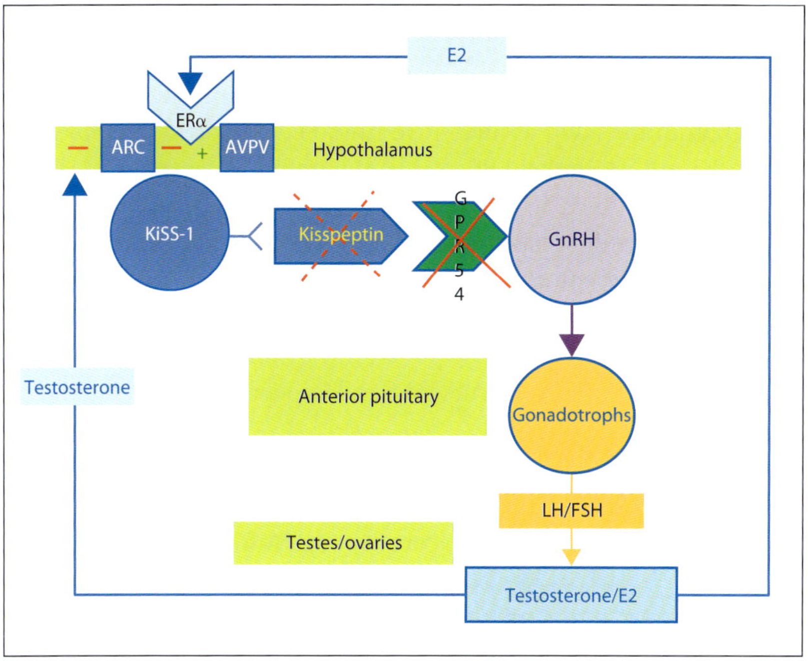

Fig. 1. Schema depicting the regulation of the HPG axis by kisspeptin signalling. Kisspeptin is a product of the *KiSS-1* gene which is highly expressed in the hypothalamic ARC, AVPV and PeN (not shown) nuclei. Kisspeptin binds to and activates its receptor GPR54 which is expressed on GnRH neurons of the MBH. The pulsatile release of GnRH from the hypothalamus stimulates the release of LH and FSH, which in turn leads to the release of gonadal sex steroids. In female rodents, oestrogen (E2) exerts a negative feedback effect on this signalling cascade at the ARC and a positive feedback effect at the AVPV. Both effects are mediated via ERα, and the latter effect on the AVPV may play a key role in the pre-ovulatory LH surge. In gonadectomised male rats, intra-ARC *KiSS-1* mRNA levels are significantly higher compared with control animals. Conversely, testosterone replacement reduces kisspeptin expression in the MBH of castrated male monkeys. Both animals and humans with mutations of GPR54 (red cross) have IHH. *KiSS-1* knockout mice (dashed red cross) exhibit a variable phenotype from complete IHH to a less severe phenotype with higher gonadal weight and more vaginal opening in the females.

hypothalamic amenorrhoea receiving twice daily kisspeptin-54 injection for 2 weeks despite the attenuation of the gonatotropin increase in response to kisspeptin [25].

Kisspeptin as a Gatekeeper of Puberty

The failure of GPR54–/– mice and humans [29, 35] and *KiSS-1*–/– mice [30] to enter puberty and the ability of kisspeptin administration to rescue the phenotype of the latter [30] suggest that kisspeptin and GPR54 play a crucial role as gatekeepers of puberty.

The ICV administration of kisspeptin-10 to juvenile male rhesus monkeys results in the precocious release of LH, an effect that is prevented by pre-treatment with a GnRH antagonist [43]. However, the ability of kisspeptin to stimulate GnRH neurons is less marked than in the adult animal. Real time-PCR has demonstrated that the expression of *KiSS-1* mRNA in the ARC of *M. mulatta* monkeys [43] and AVPV of mice [44] increases as the animals progress from the juvenile stage of development into puberty. In addition, dual-labelling studies co-localising kisspeptin-10 and GnRH have shown that the apposition of kisspeptin and GnRH neurons, first detectable at postnatal day 25 increases with progression towards puberty [4]. This is in keeping with the development of precocious puberty in a child with a GPR54 activating mutation [45]. These data strongly suggest that kisspeptin is vital for pubertal development.

Kisspeptin Expression May Be a Link between Fertility and Nutritional Status

Hypogonadotropic hypogonadism is seen in humans and *ob/ob* mice with genetic leptin deficiency [46, 47] and in humans with hypoleptinaemia as a consequence of low body weight. In these subjects, the hypogonadism can be corrected by the administration of leptin [48, 49]. The leptin receptor is expressed on kisspeptin neurons and the expression of *KiSS-1* mRNA is reduced in *ob/ob* mice but can be increased by leptin administration [50]. Kisspeptin may therefore act as a CNS mediator linking nutritional status with reproduction.

Further evidence for this comes from the relationship between kisspeptin expression in the hypothalamus and the well-established mediators of hypothalamic energy homeostasis, α-melanocyte stimulating hormone (α-MSH) and melanin-concentrating hormone (MCH) and the mammalian target of rapamycin (mTOR) which acts as a sensor of intra-cellular energy levels. α-MSH is an anorectic peptide synthesised and released by neurons of the ARC. Expression of α-MSH is highest during fasting, and levels fall when nutrition is replete [51]. ICV administration of a melanocortin agonist to ewes during the luteal phase results in an increase in *KiSS-1* mRNA in the preoptic area of the hypothalamus, a reduction in *KiSS-1* mRNA in the ARC and an increase in plasma LH [52]. Conversely, the orexigenic peptide MCH which shows high hypothalamic expression during fasting inhibits the activation of GnRH neurons by kisspeptin [53]. Lastly, the activation of mTOR by ICV administration of L-leucine to female peri-pubertal rats results in a rise in plasma LH [54]. When mTOR activation is blocked by rapamycin, the expression of *KiSS-1* mRNA in the ARC becomes almost undetectable and plasma levels of LH fall, an effect that has been shown not to be due to changes in GnRH neurons [54]. In sum, these findings may imply that the downregulation of the HPG axis which occurs in states of negative energy balance may in part be regulated by kisspeptin and that the replenishment of nutrition is permissive to kisspeptin stimulation of GnRH release.

Conclusions

Kisspeptin and GPR54 play an important role in the onset of puberty and the regulation of the HPG axis. In both human and animal models, a lack of kisspeptin signalling leads to IHH (fig. 1). Further work on kisspeptin will undoubtedly improve our understanding of the pathophysiology of this condition.

Acknowledgements

S.H. is a Medical Research Council Clinical Research Training Fellow. W.S.D. is funded by a Department of Health Clinician Scientist Award. The Department is funded by a Wellcome Trust, Medical Research Council Program Grant, the EU 6th Framework Programme DIABESITY (LSHM-CT-2003-503041), an Integrative Mammalian Biology Capacity Building Award and funding from the NIHR Biomedical Research Centre Funding Scheme.

References

1 Lee JH, Miele ME, Hicks DJ, Phillips KK, Trent JM, Weissman BE, Welch DR: KiSS-1, a novel human malignant melanoma metastasis-suppressor gene. J Natl Cancer Inst 1996;88:1731–1737.

2 Ohtaki T, Shintani Y, Honda S, Matsumoto H, Hori A, Kanehashi K, Terao Y, Kumano S, Takatsu Y, Masuda Y, Ishibashi Y, Watanabe T, Asada M, Yamada T, Suenaga M, Kitada C, Usuki S, Kurokawa T, Onda H, Nishimura O, Fujino M: Metastasis suppressor gene KiSS-1 encodes peptide ligand of a G-protein-coupled receptor. Nature 2001;411:613–617.

3 Gottsch ML, Cunningham MJ, Smith JT, Popa SM, Acohido BV, Crowley WF, Seminara S, Clifton DK, Steiner RA: A role for kisspeptins in the regulation of gonadotropin secretion in the mouse. Endocrinology 2004;145:4073–4077.

4 Clarkson J, Herbison AE: Postnatal development of kisspeptin neurons in mouse hypothalamus; sexual dimorphism and projections to gonadotropin-releasing hormone neurons. Endocrinology 2006; 147:5817–5825.

5 Richard N, Galmiche G, Corvaisier S, Caraty A, Kottler ML: KiSS-1 and GPR54 genes are co-expressed in rat gonadotrophs and differentially regulated in vivo by oestradiol and gonadotrophin-releasing hormone. J Neuroendocrinol 2008;20:381–393.

6 Muir AI, Chamberlain L, Elshourbagy NA, Michalovich D, Moore DJ, Calamari A, Szekeres PG, Sarau HM, Chambers JK, Murdock P, Steplewski K, Shabon U, Miller JE, Middleton SE, Darker JG, Larminie CG, Wilson S, Bergsma DJ, Emson P, Faull R, Philpott KL, Harrison DC: AXOR12, a novel human G protein-coupled receptor, activated by the peptide KiSS-1. J Biol Chem 2001;276:28969–28975.

7 Kotani M, Detheux M, Vandenbogaerde A, Communi D, Vanderwinden JM, Le PE, Brezillon S, Tyldesley R, Suarez-Huerta N, Vandeput F, Blanpain C, Schiffmann SN, Vassart G, Parmentier M: The metastasis suppressor gene KiSS-1 encodes kisspeptins, the natural ligands of the orphan G protein-coupled receptor GPR54. J Biol Chem 2001;276:34631–34636.

8 Clements MK, McDonald TP, Wang R, Xie G, O'Dowd BF, George SR, Austin CP, Liu Q: FMRFamide-related neuropeptides are agonists of the orphan G-protein-coupled receptor GPR54. Biochem Biophys Res Commun 2001;284:1189–1193.

9 Lee DK, Nguyen T, O'Neill GP, Cheng R, Liu Y, Howard AD, Coulombe N, Tan CP, Tang-Nguyen AT, George SR, O'Dowd BF: Discovery of a receptor related to the galanin receptors. FEBS Lett 1999;446: 103–107.

10 Robin-Jagerschmidt C, Sylte I, Bihoreau C, Hendricksen L, Calvet A, Dahl SG, Benicourt C: The ligand binding site of NPY at the rat Y1 receptor investigated by site-directed mutagenesis and molecular modeling. Mol Cell Endocrinol 1998:139: 187–198.

11 Messager S, Chatzidaki EE, Ma D, Hendrick AG, Zahn D, Dixon J, Thresher RR, Malinge I, Lomet D, Carlton MB, Colledge WH, Caraty A, Aparicio SA: Kisspeptin directly stimulates gonadotropin-releasing hormone release via G protein-coupled receptor 54. Proc Natl Acad Sci USA 2005;102:1761–1766.
12 Silverman AJ, Antunes JL, Ferin M, Zimmerman EA: The distribution of luteinizing hormone-releasing hormone (LHRH) in the hypothalamus of the rhesus monkey. Light microscopic studies using immunoperoxidase technique. Endocrinology 1977; 101:134–142.
13 Silverman AJ, Wilson R, Kesner JS, Knobil E: Hypothalamic localization of multiunit electrical activity associated with pulsatile LH release in the rhesus monkey. Neuroendocrinology 1986;44:168–171.
14 Plant TM, Krey LC, Moossy J, McCormack JT, Hess DL, Knobil E: The arcuate nucleus and the control of gonadotropin and prolactin secretion in the female rhesus monkey *(Macaca mulatta)*. Endocrinology 1978;102:52–62.
15 Navarro VM, Castellano JM, Fernandez-Fernandez R, Tovar S, Roa J, Mayen A, Nogueiras R, Vazquez MJ, Barreiro ML, Magni P, Aguilar E, Dieguez C, Pinilla L, Tena-Sempere M: Characterization of the potent luteinizing hormone-releasing activity of KiSS-1 peptide, the natural ligand of GPR54. Endocrinology 2005;146:156–163.
16 Thompson EL, Patterson M, Murphy KG, Smith KL, Dhillo WS, Todd JF, Ghatei MA, Bloom SR: Central and peripheral administration of kisspeptin-10 stimulates the hypothalamic-pituitary-gonadal axis. J Neuroendocrinol 2004;16:850–858.
17 Liu X, Lee K, Herbison AE: Kisspeptin excites gonadotropin-releasing hormone neurons through a phospholipase C/calcium-dependent pathway regulating multiple ion channels. Endocrinology 2008;149:4605–4614.
18 Sagar SM, Sharp FR, Curran T: Expression of c-fos protein in brain: metabolic mapping at the cellular level. Science 1988;240:1328–1331.
19 Hewson AK, Dickson SL: Systemic administration of ghrelin induces Fos and Egr-1 proteins in the hypothalamic arcuate nucleus of fasted and fed rats. J Neuroendocrinol 2000;12:1047–1049.
20 Irwig MS, Fraley GS, Smith JT, Acohido BV, Popa SM, Cunningham MJ, Gottsch ML, Clifton DK, Steiner RA: Kisspeptin activation of gonadotropin releasing hormone neurons and regulation of KiSS-1 mRNA in the male rat. Neuroendocrinology 2004; 80:264–72.
21 Roseweir AK, Kauffman AS, Smith JT, Guerriero KA, Morgan K, Pielecka-Fortuna J, Pineda R, Gottsch ML, Tena-Sempere M, Moenter SM, Terasawa E, Clarke IJ, Steiner RA, Millar RP: Discovery of potent kisspeptin antagonists delineate physiological mechanisms of gonadotropin regulation. J Neurosci 2009; 29:3920–3929.
22 Clarkson J, d'Anglemont de Tassingny X, Moreno AS, Colledge WH, Herbison AE: Kisspeptin-GPR54 signaling is essential for preovulatory gonadotropin-releasing hormone neuron activation and the luteinizing hormone surge. J Neurosci 2008;28:8691–8697.
23 Dhillo WS, Chaudhri OB, Patterson M, Thompson EL, Murphy KG, Badman MK, McGowan BM, Amber V, Patel S, Ghatei MA, Bloom SR: Kisspeptin-54 stimulates the hypothalamic-pituitary gonadal axis in human males. J Clin Endocrinol Metab 2005;90:6609–6615.
24 Dhillo WS, Chaudhri OB, Thompson EL, Murphy KG, Patterson M, Ramachandran R, Nijher GK, Amber V, Kokkinos A, Donaldson M, Ghatei MA, Bloom SR: Kisspeptin-54 stimulates gonadotropin release most potently during the preovulatory phase of the menstrual cycle in women. J Clin Endocrinol Metab 2007;92:3958–3966.
25 Jayasena CN, Nijher GM, Chaudhri OB, Murphy KG, Ranger A, Lim A, Patel D, Mehta A, Todd C, Ramachandran R, Salem V, Stamp GW, Donaldson M, Ghatei MA, Bloom SR, Dhillo WS: Subcutaneous injection of kisspeptin-54 acutely stimulates gonadotropin secretion in women with hypothalamic amenorrhea, but chronic administration causes tachyphylaxis. J Clin Endocrinol Metab 2009;94:4315–4323.
26 Lee JH, Welch DR: Suppression of metastasis in human breast carcinoma MDA-MB-435 cells after transfection with the metastasis suppressor gene, KiSS-1. Cancer Res 1997;57:2384–2387.
27 Franco B, Guioli S, Pragliola A, Incerti B, Bardoni B, Tonlorenzi R, Carrozzo R, Maestrini E, Pieretti M, Taillon-Miller P: A gene deleted in Kallmann's syndrome shares homology with neural cell adhesion and axonal path-finding molecules. Nature 1991; 353:529–536.
28 Legouis R, Hardelin JP, Levilliers J, Claverie JM, Compain S, Wunderle V, Millasseau P, Le PD, Cohen D, Caterina D: The candidate gene for the X-linked Kallmann syndrome encodes a protein related to adhesion molecules. Cell 1991;67:423–435.
29 de Roux N, Genin E, Carel JC, Matsuda F, Chaussain JL, Milgrom E: Hypogonadotropic hypogonadism due to loss of function of the KiSS1-derived peptide receptor GPR54. Proc Natl Acad Sci USA 2003;100: 10972–10976.

30 d'Anglemont de Tassigny X, Fagg LA, Dixon JP, Day K, Leitch HG, Hendrick AG, Zahn D, Franceschini I, Caraty A, Carlton MB, Aparicio SA, Colledge WH: Hypogonadotropic hypogonadism in mice lacking a functional Kiss1 gene. Proc Natl Acad Sci USA 2007;104:10714–10719.

31 Lapatto R, Pallais JC, Zhang D, Chan YM, Mahan A, Cerrato F, Le WW, Hoffman GE, Seminara SB: Kiss1–/– mice exhibit more variable hypogonadism than Gpr54–/– mice. Endocrinology 2007;148:4927–4936.

32 Gutierrez-Pascual E, Martínez-Fuentes AJ, Pinilla L, Tena-Sempere M, Malagon MM, Castano JP: Direct pituitary effects of kisspeptin: activation of gonadotrophs and somatotrophs and stimulation of luteinising hormone and growth hormone secretion. J Neuroendocrinol 2007;19:521–530.

33 Smith JT, Rao A, Pereira A, Caraty A, Millar RP, Clarke IJ: Kisspeptin is present in ovine hypophysial portal blood but does not increase during the preovulatory luteinizing hormone surge: evidence that gonadotropes are not direct targets of kisspeptin in vivo. Endocrinology 2008;149:1951–1959.

34 Plant TM, Ramaswamy S, Dipietro MJ: Repetitive activation of hypothalamic G protein-coupled receptor 54 with intravenous pulses of kisspeptin in the juvenile monkey *(Macaca mulatta)* elicits a sustained train of gonadotropin-releasing hormone discharges. Endocrinology 2006;147:1007–1013.

35 Seminara SB, Messager S, Chatzidaki EE, Thresher RR, Acierno JS Jr, Shagoury JK, Bo-Abbas Y, Kuohung W, Schwinof KM, Hendrick AG, Zahn D, Dixon J, Kaiser UB, Slaugenhaupt SA, Gusella JF, O'Rahilly S, Carlton MB, Crowley WF Jr, Aparicio SA, Colledge WH: The GPR54 gene as a regulator of puberty. N Engl J Med 2003;349:1614–1627.

36 Wintermantel TM, Campbell RE, Porteous R, Bock D, Grone HJ, Todman MG, Korach KS, Greiner E, Perez CA, Schutz G, Herbison AE: Definition of estrogen receptor pathway critical for estrogen positive feedback to gonadotropin-releasing hormone neurons and fertility. Neuron 2006;52:271–280.

37 Hrabovszky E, Shughrue PJ, Merchenthaler I, Hajszan T, Carpenter CD, Liposits Z, Petersen SL: Detection of estrogen receptor-beta messenger ribonucleic acid and 125I-estrogen binding sites in luteinizing hormone-releasing hormone neurons of the rat brain. Endocrinology 2000;141:3506–3509.

38 Smith JT, Cunningham MJ, Rissman EF, Clifton DK, Steiner RA: Regulation of Kiss1 gene expression in the brain of the female mouse. Endocrinology 2005;146:3686–3692.

39 Adachi S, Yamada S, Takatsu Y, Matsui H, Kinoshita M, Takase K, Sugiura H, Ohtaki T, Matsumoto H, Uenoyama Y, Tsukamura H, Inoue K, Maeda K: Involvement of anteroventral periventricular metastin/kisspeptin neurons in estrogen positive feedback action on luteinizing hormone release in female rats. J Reprod Dev 2007;53:367–378.

40 Shibata M, Friedman RL, Ramaswamy S, Plant TM: Evidence that down regulation of hypothalamic KiSS-1 expression is involved in the negative feedback action of testosterone to regulate luteinising hormone secretion in the adult male rhesus monkey *(Macaca mulatta)*. J Neuroendocrinol 2007;19:432–438.

41 Seminara SB, Dipietro MJ, Ramaswamy S, Crowley WF Jr, Plant TM: Continuous human metastin 45–54 infusion desensitizes G protein-coupled receptor 54-induced gonadotropin-releasing hormone release monitored indirectly in the juvenile male Rhesus monkey *(Macaca mulatta)*: a finding with therapeutic implications. Endocrinology 2006;147:2122–2126.

42 Belchetz PE, Plant TM, Nakai Y, Keogh EJ, Knobil E: Hypophysial responses to continuous and intermittent delivery of hypopthalamic gonadotropin-releasing hormone. Science 1978;202:631–633.

43 Shahab M, Mastronardi C, Seminara SB, Crowley WF, Ojeda SR, Plant TM: Increased hypothalamic GPR54 signaling: a potential mechanism for initiation of puberty in primates. Proc Natl Acad Sci USA 2005;102:2129–2134.

44 Han SK, Gottsch ML, Lee KJ, Popa SM, Smith JT, Jakawich SK, Clifton DK, Steiner RA, Herbison AE: Activation of gonadotropin-releasing hormone neurons by kisspeptin as a neuroendocrine switch for the onset of puberty. J Neurosci 2005;25:11349–11356.

45 Teles MG, Bianco SD, Brito VN, Trarbach EB, Kuohung W, Xu S, Seminara SB, Mendonca BB, Kaiser UB, Latronico AC: A GPR54-activating mutation in a patient with central precocious puberty. N Engl J Med 2008;358:709–715.

46 Coleman DL: Obese and diabetes: two mutant genes causing diabetes-obesity syndromes in mice. Diabetologia 1978;14:141–148.

47 Clément K, Vaisse C, Lahlou N, Cabrol S, Pelloux V, Cassuto D, Gourmelen M, Dina C, Chambaz J, Lacorte JM, Basdevant A, Bougneres P, Lebouc Y, Froguel P, Guy-Grand B: A mutation in the human leptin receptor gene causes obesity and pituitary dysfunction. Nature 1998;392:398–401.

48 Welt CK, Chan JL, Bullen J, Murphy R, Smith P, DePaoli AM, Karalis A, Mantzoros CS: Recombinant human leptin in women with hypothalamic amenorrhea. N Engl J Med 2004;351:987–997.

49 Farooqi IS, Jebb SA, Langmack G, Lawrence E, Cheetham CH, Prentice AM, Hughes IA, McCamish MA, O'Rahilly S: Effects of recombinant leptin therapy in a child with congenital leptin deficiency. N Engl J Med 1999341:879–884.
50 Smith JT, Acohido BV, Clifton DK, Steiner RA: KiSS-1 neurones are direct targets for leptin in the ob/ob mouse. J Neuroendocrinol 2006;18:298–303.
51 Mizuno TM, Kleopoulos SP, Bergen HT, Roberts JL, Priest CA, Mobbs CV: Hypothalamic pro-opiomelanocortin mRNA is reduced by fasting and [corrected] in ob/ob and db/db mice, but is stimulated by leptin. Diabetes 1998;47:294–297.
52 Backholer K, Smith J, Clarke IJ: Melanocortins may stimulate reproduction by activating orexin neurons in the dorsomedial hypothalamus and kisspeptin neurons in the preoptic area of the ewe. Endocrinology 2009, Epub ahead of print.
53 Wu M, Dumalska I, Morozova E, van den PA, Alreja M: Melanin-concentrating hormone directly inhibits GnRH neurons and blocks kisspeptin activation, linking energy balance to reproduction. Proc Natl Acad Sci USA 2009;106:17217–17222.
54 Roa J, Garcia-Galiano D, Varela L, Sanchez-Garrido MA, Pineda R, Castellano JM, Ruiz-Pino F, Romero M, Aguilar E, Lopez M, Gaytan F, Dieguez C, Pinilla L, Tena-Sempere M: The mammalian target of rapamycin as novel central regulator of puberty onset via modulation of hypothalamic Kiss1 system. Endocrinology 2009;150:5016–5026.

Waljit S. Dhillo, PhD, FRCPath, FRCP
Reader in Endocrinology and Metabolism
Section of Investigative Medicine, Faculty of Medicine, Imperial College London
6th Floor Commonwealth Building, Hammersmith Hospital
Du Cane Road, London W12 OHS (UK)
Tel. +44 208 383 2820, Fax +44 208 383 8320, E-Mail w.dhillo@imperial.ac.uk

Quinton R (ed): Kallmann Syndrome and Hypogonadotropic Hypogonadism.
Front Horm Res. Basel, Karger, 2010, vol 39, pp 37–50

Role of Fibroblast Growth Factor Signaling in Gonadotropin-Releasing Hormone Neuronal System Development

Wilson C.J. Chung · Pei-San Tsai

Department of Integrative Physiology and Center for Neuroscience, University of Colorado at Boulder, Boulder, Colo., USA

Abstract

There is growing evidence demonstrating that fibroblast growth factor (FGF) signaling is important for the development of the gonadotropin-releasing hormone (GnRH) neuronal system. In humans, loss-of-function mutations in FGF receptor 1 *(Fgfr1)* and *Fgf8* lead to hypogonadotropic hypogonadism (HH) with or without anosmia. Insights into how FGF signaling deficiency disrupts the GnRH system in humans are beginning to emerge from studies using transgenic mouse models. In this review, we summarize GnRH system defects in several lines of FGF signaling-deficient mice. We showed that FGF signaling is critically required for olfactory placode induction, differentiation, and GnRH neuronal fate specification and postnatal maintenance. Extrapolating from these transgenic mouse data, we suggest that idiopathic HH in patients harboring loss-of-function *Fgfr1* and/or *Fgf8* mutations is not merely a result of defective GnRH neuronal migration, but also insults accumulated in the GnRH system during fate specification and postnatal development.

Gonadotropin-releasing hormone (GnRH) neurons are central to reproductive function in all vertebrates. Unlike most neurons in the brain, GnRH neurons are not born within the central nervous system (CNS) [1, 2]. Although the origin of GnRH neurons in non-mammalian species is still under debate [3, 4], the consensus in mammals is that GnRH neurons emerge from the olfactory placode during early embryogenesis and subsequently migrate across the cribriform plate to enter the forebrain. Once migration ceases, GnRH neurons target their axons to the external zone of the median eminence (ME) for hormone release [5]. Thus, the formation of the GnRH system during development requires the entrance of GnRH neurons into three distinct developmental phases including fate specification, migration, and axon targeting. Since the disruption of any of these developmental phases could lead to an aberrantly formed GnRH system and reproductive impairment, each developmental phase must be intricately regulated.

In 1995, we identified fibroblast growth factors (FGFs) as potent neurotrophic regulators of immortalized GT1 GnRH neuronal cell lines [6] and hypothesized that the disruption of FGF signaling could be an underlying cause for human reproductive impairment. This prediction later came true when FGF receptor 1 *(Fgfr1)* was identified as a causal gene underlying an autosomal dominant form of Kallmann syndrome (KS) [7], a human disorder characterized by hypogonadotropic hypogonadism (HH) and anosmia. A few years later, Pitteloud et al. [8, 9] showed that loss-of-function *Fgfr1* mutations also caused idiopathic HH (IHH) in normosmic individuals, reaffirming a strong relationship between FGF signaling and function of the GnRH system. Most recently, Falardeau et al. [10] demonstrated that mutations in one of the FGF ligands, *Fgf8*, could underlie varying degrees of IHH with or without anosmia. Of note, although these human studies revealed an important link between FGF signaling and function of the GnRH system, it is unclear whether FGF signaling deficiency alters genesis, migration, or axon targeting of developing GnRH neurons, or if they lead to a postnatal dysfunction of the GnRH system. At the mechanistic level, these questions are very difficult to answer in humans. To circumvent this problem, investigations using mouse models deficient in various components of FGF signaling have been launched.

The development of GnRH neurons in mice has been extensively characterized. The olfactory placodes in mice develop from the anterior neural ridge [11] as the ventrolateral ectodermal thickenings. At embryonic day 10 (E10), the placode invaginates to form the olfactory pit, which invaginates again to form a secondary medial recess after 12 h. GnRH neurons (defined by the production of GnRH) are first seen in the medial olfactory pit at about E11.0–E11.5 [1, 12]. After fate specification, GnRH neurons begin an en masse migration at E11.5 to enter the forebrain. The migration of GnRH neurons in the nasal cavity is guided by the peripherin-positive tracts of the vomeronasal (VNN) and olfactory nerve [13]. By E14.5, the majority of GnRH neurons have crossed the nasal-brain junction. After reaching the forebrain, GnRH neurons make a ventral turn to follow a subset of peripherin-positive fibers to reach their final destinations [14]. At this time, a portion of GnRH neurons begins to extend their axons to the ME [15–17]. By E16, a network of GnRH neurons can be observed in a bilateral continuum from the base of the olfactory bulbs to the ME, and the formation of the GnRH neuronal system is largely complete.

To date, a long list of transcription factors, guidance molecules, neurotransmitters, cell surface molecules, growth factors, and receptors have been shown to regulate distinct phases of GnRH neuronal development in the mouse [18, 19]. This list speaks to the impressive redundancy involved in the formation of a critical neuroendocrine system. The pressing questions are, then, which regulators are (1) truly indispensable and (2) bear significant clinical relevance to human GnRH system defects? Compelling evidence now places FGF signaling as a prime candidate that is both indispensable and clinically relevant to the formation and maintenance of GnRH neurons. The goal of the present review is to provide an overview of GnRH system defects in transgenic

Table 1. List of transgenic mice deficient in FGF signaling used in our studies

Name of mouse	Deficiency syndrome	Utility of mouse model	Limitations of model
dnFGFR	Disrupts functions of FGFRs 1, 2 and 3 specifically in GnRH neurons	Study tissue-specific effects of attenuated FGF signaling on later phases of GnRH neuronal migration, axon targeting and postnatal function.	(1) Not appropriate for studying GnRH neuronal fate specification and early migration. (2) The extent of FGFR function disruption depends on the activity of the GnRH promoter. (3) Does not reveal which component of FGF signaling is involved.
Fgfr3 KO	Global deletion of functional FGFR3 protein.	Study effects of global deletion of FGFR3 on GnRH system development and postnatal function.	Not tissue specific, but appropriate for examining *all* stages of pre-/post- natal GnRH system development.
Fgf8 hypomorph	Global reduction of functional FGF8 protein due to a splicing defect caused by neo-cassette insertion.	Study effects of global reduction of FGF8 on GnRH system development and postnatal function.	Not tissue specific, but appropriate for examining *all* stages of pre-/post- natal GnRH system development.
Fgfr1 hypomorph	Global reduction in functional FGFR1 protein due to a splicing defect caused by neo-cassette insertion	Study effects of global reduction in FGFR1 on GnRH system development and postnatal function.	Not tissue specific, but appropriate for examining *all* stages of pre-/post- natal GnRH system development.

mice deficient in various components of FGF signaling. By doing so, we will answer two important questions. First, which FGF ligand(s) and receptor(s) critically regulate GnRH neuronal development? Second, which phase(s) of GnRH neuronal development (fate specification, migration, or axon targeting) is severely impacted by FGF signaling deficiency? Extrapolating from the mouse studies, we hope to shed light on how FGF signaling components interact in a time-dependent fashion to support the development and maintenance of the human GnRH system.

Transgenic Mouse Models

This review will analyze GnRH system defects in four lines of transgenic mice deficient in FGF signaling. Each transgenic mouse line provides a unique tool for disrupting FGF signaling, but also has its own limitations (table 1).

A transgenic mouse (dnFGFR mouse) was generated by targeting the expression of a dominant-negative FGFR (dnFGFR) to GnRH neurons using the rat GnRH promoter [20]. Although this mouse allows the tissue-specific disruption of FGFR function in GnRH neurons, it comes with two limitations. First, it is not suitable for studying the very early phase of GnRH neuronal development (including fate specification) because GnRH promoter activity at this early period is presumably too weak to drive the expression of dnFGFR. Second, since dnFGFR disrupts the function of FGFRs 1, 2, and 3 [20], the observed phenotypes cannot be attributed to the disruption of a specific FGFR subtype. To circumvent these limitations, we utilize mice that are hypomorphic for *Fgfr1* (*Fgfr1* hypomorphs) [21] and knockout for *Fgfr3* (*Fgfr3* KO) [22] to elucidate the contribution of each receptor and to ensure their deficiency/deletion at the very beginning of GnRH neuron genesis. The reasons for concentrating on these two FGFRs are described in the section below. Since FGF8 has been identified as an FGF ligand indispensable for the morphogenesis of the olfactory region [23], the birthplace of GnRH neurons, we also use mice hypomorphic for *Fgf8* (*Fgf8* hypomorphs) to examine the specific contribution of this ligand. It is important to note that *Fgfr1* hypomorphs, *Fgf8* hypomorphs, and *Fgfr3* KO bear the global deletion/deficiency in FGF signaling components; thus, indirect effects upon GnRH neurons cannot be ruled out. However, compared to mice with tissue-specific disruption, the hemizygous state of global disruption in these mice may be more comparable to humans harboring *Fgfr1* and/or *Fgf8* mutations.

Regulation of Gonadotropin-Releasing Hormone Neuronal Fate Specification by Fibroblast Growth Factor Signaling

Landmark studies showed that the vast majority (~80%) of mouse GnRH neurons undergo their last division in the olfactory placode between E9.5 and E10.5 [2]. Interestingly, these postmitotic olfactory placode progenitor cells do not express detectable levels of GnRH mRNA or peptide prior to E11.5 [1, 2]. In this sense, one can define the period of GnRH neuron fate specification to occur between E9.5–E11.5. The absence of measurable GnRH peptide prior to E11.5 is a major hurdle for studying the molecular processes that regulate GnRH neuronal fate specification, because at present the only marker for GnRH neurons is GnRH itself. Therefore, postmitotic olfactory placode progenitor cells that are destined to become GnRH neurons cannot be identified during a large portion of the fate specification, before they express measurable GnRH levels. Notwithstanding this major caveat, our laboratory has accumulated mounting evidence that the activation of FGF signaling is important for the fate specification of the mouse GnRH neuronal system.

In mice, FGF signaling is mediated by four specific types of FGFRs [24]. Localization studies from our laboratory showed that the E10.5 mouse olfactory placode contained abundant levels of FGFR1, FGFR2 and FGFR3, but not FGFR4 protein

[25]. Furthermore, dual immunocytochemistry detected the presence of FGFR1 and FGFR3, but not FGFR2 protein in E15.5 and postnatal-day-3 GnRH neurons [25]. This is consistent with an earlier observation showing that *Fgfr1* and *Fgfr3* mRNA is expressed in immortalized mouse GnRH neuronal cell lines [6]. The strongest data indicating that FGF signaling plays a role in GnRH neuronal fate specification are derived from in vitro nasal explants isolated from E10.5 embryos. In this experimental paradigm, the number of GnRH neurons in the nasal explants increased after 2 or 3 days in vitro [25]. This increase in GnRH neurons was inhibited by the FGFR antagonist SU5402, indicating the activation of FGFR is required for GnRH neuron fate specification [25].

The aforementioned studies provided the impetus for identifying the specific FGF signaling component(s) required for GnRH neuronal fate specification. Based on the presence of FGFR1 and FGFR3 in GnRH neurons, we hypothesized that activation of these receptors was critical for mouse GnRH neuronal fate specification. Therefore, disruption of FGFR1 or FGFR3 function is expected to result in a defective GnRH neuronal system. We tested this hypothesis using mice globally deficient in FGFR1 (*Fgfr1* hypomorphs) or FGFR3 (*Fgfr3* KO), which have a major advantage. Unlikely tissue-specific KOs that require the GnRH promoter to be active before disruption can occur, the global disruption of genes guarantees FGFR1 or FGFR3 deficiency at the time of GnRH neuronal fate specification. We first examined the total number of GnRH neurons in the entire heads of newborn wild-type, heterozygous and homozygous *Fgfr1* hypomorphs, and found that the number of GnRH neurons in homozygous *Fgfr1* hypomorphs was about 88% lower than their wild-type littermates [26]. Furthermore, there was no significant difference between heterozygous *Fgfr1* hypomorphs and their wild-type littermates [26]. On the other hand, the number of GnRH neurons was unaffected in newborn *Fgfr3* KO mice [26]. These whole animal studies corroborated the nasal explant studies and supported the idea that activation of FGFR function may be a key pathway required for the emergence of GnRH neurons [25]. Furthermore, by comparing the GnRH neuronal system between *Fgfr1* hypomorphic and *Fgfr3* KO mice, we established that the activation of FGFR1, but not FGFR3, is required for the normal number of GnRH neurons in the newborn mouse head.

Of the 22 identified FGF ligands, there are several lines of experimentally derived evidence indicating that FGF8 is the most likely FGF candidate to be involved in the early development of GnRH neurons. First, *Fgf8* mRNA is found in the ectodermal region ventral/lateral of the telencephalic commissural plate on E9.5, which will form the olfactory placode [23, 27]. This expression profile suggests that FGF8 signaling is critically important for the induction and differentiation of the mouse olfactory placode. Second, a partial loss of FGF8 function resulted in the absence of the olfactory bulbs and vomeronasal organs (VNO) [26, 28]. The absence of the VNO has a special relevance given that the VNO also originates in the olfactory placode [2]. Third, FGF8 has been shown to bind and readily activate FGFR signaling, including FGFR1, in cell lines [10]. Therefore, we hypothesized that disruption of FGF8 signaling will severely impair the genesis of the GnRH neuronal system. To test this hypothesis, we examined the GnRH neuronal system in newborn *Fgf8* hypomorphic mice, which in the homozygous state shows a ~54% downregulation of *Fgf8* mRNA [28]. Much to our surprise, the GnRH neuronal system in homozygous *Fgf8* hypomorphs was not partially affected, but eliminated in its entirety [10, 26]. An equally striking observation was that heterozygous *Fgf8* hypomorphs had approximately 50% fewer GnRH neurons remaining as compared to wild-type littermates [10, 26]. These results led to our conclusion that the prenatal development of the mouse GnRH neuronal system is extremely dependent on the presence of FGFR1 and FGF8 signaling.

A major constraint of studies in newborn mice mentioned before is that they do not elucidate whether FGF8 signaling is required for GnRH neuronal fate specification or other developmental processes, such as neuronal survival after emergence. Therefore, we expanded our studies to include the analysis of the E11.5 GnRH neuronal system, when GnRH neurons are first detectable using immunocytochemistry. By examining the emergence of GnRH neurons from the E11.5 olfactory placode, we were able to directly answer the question: Is FGF8 signaling required for the fate specification process of GnRH neurons in the olfactory placode? In contrast to wild-type embryos, we did not detect any GnRH neurons in the olfactory placode of homozygous *Fgf8* hypomorphs on E11.5 or in any subsequent time points that were examined [26]. Together with the previously described nasal explant studies, these data strongly suggest that FGF8 signaling acting through FGFR1 is critical for GnRH neuron fate specification in the mouse olfactory placode.

Interestingly, we found that the secondary recess of the E11.5 olfactory placode from where GnRH neurons emerge is virtually absent in homozygous *Fgf8* hypomorphs. The dysgenesis of this secondary recess is likely the underlying cause for the failure of GnRH neurons to emerge (fig. 1). Our preliminary data showing that the VNO is missing in the homozygous *Fgf8* hypomorphs are consistent with the notion that this recess fails to develop and give rise to differentiated derivatives. Our data also suggest the presence of discrete developmental zones in the olfactory placode [13], with FGF8 signaling deficiency more likely to impact the zone that gives rise to the epithelial cells of the VNO and GnRH neurons. Currently, we are studying how a partial loss of FGF8 function could severely disrupt the developmental organization of the secondary recess of the olfactory placode.

Regulation of Gonadotropin-Releasing Hormone Neuron Migration by Fibroblast Growth Factor Signaling

The organization and functionality of the GnRH neuronal system depends not only on the proper emergence of GnRH neurons from the olfactory placode, but also on the accurate migration from the olfactory placode to the preoptic/hypothalamus

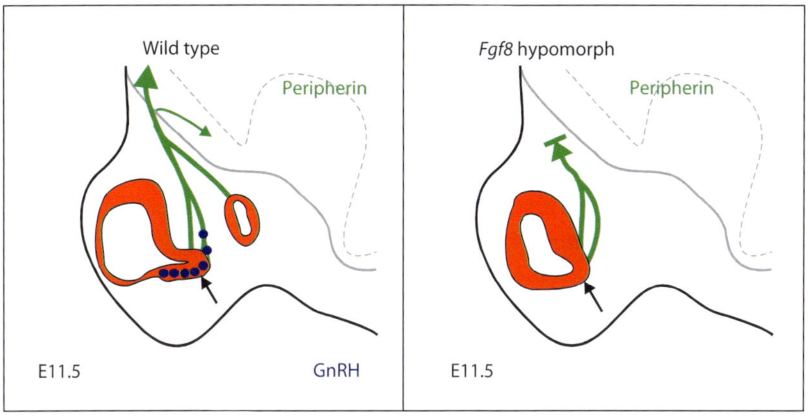

Fig. 1. Parasagittal schematic representation of the mouse olfactory placode (red) on E11.5. The secondary recess (arrow) in the olfactory placode, from where the GnRH neurons (blue) emerge, is present in the wild-type, but not in the homozygous *Fgf8* hypomorphic embryo. This suggests that the formation of this recess is FGF8 dependent. FGF8 signaling is also important for the development of the peripherin-positive fibers (green) of the VNN, which fail to enter the homozygous *Fgf8* hypomorphic mouse forebrain. However, because GnRH neurons were eliminated prior to entering the migrational phase, we hypothesize that the primary impact of FGF8 deficiency is upon the fate specification process of GnRH neurons.

region. Indeed, the failure of GnRH neurons to migrate and transition from the nasal cavity into the anterior forebrain was considered to be the major cause of GnRH deficiency in KS [29]. This view was based on the observation that GnRH migration was arrested just prior to entering the forebrain in a 19-week-old fetus with the X-linked form of KS [30]. Indeed, no GnRH neurons were detected in the forebrain regions where they were expected during this stage of embryonic development, but were instead found beneath the forebrain within the meninges [29]. Moreover, the VNN fibers in this KS fetus also ended within the meninges and failed to contact the developing olfactory bulbs [29].

GnRH migratory defect is frequently extrapolated to be the key cause of IHH in all forms of KS, including KS patients who harbor loss-of-function mutations in the *Fgfr1* or *Fgf8* genes [7, 10]. It is possible that GnRH migration is affected in these KS patients, but there are no studies verifying this in human fetuses with mutations in *Fgfr1* or *Fgf8*. In fact, mouse studies done in our laboratory found little evidence supporting the view that defects in FGF signaling cause impaired GnRH neuronal migration. Only a slight arrest (<10%) in GnRH neurons was detected in the intrahemispheric area of newborn dnFGFR mice as compared to their wild-type counterparts [31]. This slight arrest in GnRH neuron migration is inconsistent with the significant reduction of GnRH neurons in the preoptic/hypothalamus of adult dnFGFR mice. The majority of GnRH neurons in dnFGFR mice still migrated normally into the brain [20], and the loss of GnRH neurons in dnFGFR mice is due primarily to postnatal disappearance instead of migratory defects. These data suggest that the disruption of FGFR function directly at the level of GnRH neurons plays only a minor role in their migration [31].

One might also question if global deficiency of FGF signaling could alter the pathfinding of axons that guide GnRH neuronal migration, thereby indirectly disrupting this migratory process. It is interesting to note that the peripherin-positive fibers of VNN were in fact disrupted and failed to target the telencephalon of homozygous *Fgf8* hypomorphs (fig. 1) [26]. However, it is important to emphasize that GnRH neurons were already missing in these transgenic mice prior to migration; thus, the cause of GnRH system defect in these mice is failure to emerge, not failure to migrate. In heterozygous *Fgf8* hypomorphs with 50% of GnRH neurons still remaining, the reduction in GnRH neurons was also not due to defective GnRH migration. We base this conclusion on our analysis of the entire head of these newborn mice, in which we did not find any evidence of abnormal accumulation of GnRH neurons along the migrational pathway prior to entering the brain [26]. A similar observation was made for homozygous *Fgfr1* hypomorphs. Consequently, data from mice suggest that IHH in KS patients harboring *Fgfr1* or *Fgf8* mutations is more likely caused by defects in GnRH neuronal fate specification than in migration.

Regulation of Gonadotropin-Releasing Hormone Axon Targeting by Fibroblast Growth Factor Signaling

During axon targeting, GnRH fibers extend ventrally in a highly directional manner to terminate upon the fenestrated capillaries within the external zone of the ME. GnRH is released into the primary capillary plexus to reach the hypothalamo-pituitary portal veins, and ultimately the anterior pituitary. Thus, this is the stage that confers final fertility. In order for GnRH axons to target the ME properly, two events must occur: (1) the extension of the axons, and (2) the directional growth of axons to the proper target. There is virtually nothing known about the mechanisms of GnRH axon targeting in humans. However, there is a wealth of information on how FGF signaling regulates GnRH axon targeting in mice.

Regarding the extension of axons, in vitro data from our laboratory showed that this process is regulated by FGF signaling [25]. The addition of FGF2, a prototypic FGF, significantly stimulated neurite outgrowth in cultured E15.5 GnRH neurons [25]. Importantly, GnRH neurons isolated from dnFGFR mouse embryos exhibited attenuated neurite outgrowth in culture [32], suggesting FGF signaling is an endogenous cue that maintains GnRH axon growth. Regarding the directional axonal growth to the proper target, Silverman et al. [33] showed that GnRH neurons grafted into the third ventricle targeted axons to the ME, and this directional axonal growth was due to the presence of a diffusible chemoattractive signal(s) in the target [34]. To date, the identity of the diffusible chemoattractant(s) remains elusive, but several lines of evidence suggest FGFs might be one of the components. FGF2, a molecule produced in abundance by both endothelial cells and ventricular tanycytes of the ME, served as a diffusible cue to attract the directional growth of GnRH axons in an organotypic culture system [35]. The caveat is that while the study showed an attractive response of GnRH axons to an exogenously added FGF, it did not verify the role of FGFs as endogenous regulators in this process. To satisfy the criterion of FGF signaling as an endogenous chemoattractive regulator, we have demonstrated that in cultured embryonic GnRH neurons, the directional outgrowth of neurites toward the cocultured ME explant is significantly reduced in GnRH neurons expressing dnFGFR [32]. Further indirect evidence arises from the recent observation that anosmin-1, the diffusible extracellular product of *KAL1*, in turn exerts a modulatory role of FGF2/FGFR1 signaling [36].

Overall, our in vitro results showed attenuated FGF signaling disrupted the ability of GnRH neurites to extend and to grow in a directional manner. Do these in vitro alterations translate into GnRH system defects in the whole animal? There is evidence that suggests they do, but these in vivo defects are somewhat less striking. GnRH neurons in dnFGFR mice showed a significant but small reduction (15%) in the uptake of peripherally injected fluorogold, a retrograde tracer, indicating compromised contact between GnRH axons and circumventricular organs such as the ME [32]. That GnRH axon targeting is only modestly disrupted in dnFGFR mice argues for the presence of other compensatory mechanisms guiding GnRH axons in vivo. Since GnRH axon targeting is a highly axophilic event in which GnRH axons travel with other growing axons [34], these guiding axons could drive the extension and directional growth of GnRH axons via physical or other FGF-independent means. Overall, despite significant defects observed in vitro, adequate GnRH fibers have targeted the ME of dnFGFR mice to support reproduction. Current evidence suggests that GnRH axon targeting in the whole animal does not appear to be a process that critically requires FGF signaling.

Regulation of Postnatal Gonadotropin-Releasing Hormone System Function by Fibroblast Growth Factor Signaling

The proper timing of pubertal onset and reproductive senescence is key to a normal reproductive lifespan. In this regard, a healthy GnRH system becomes activated in a timely fashion and remains functional for a period of time optimal for the propagation of offspring. At present, there is direct and circumstantial evidence for a role of FGF signaling in the onset and termination of the mouse GnRH system function, thereby determining the duration of the reproductive lifespan.

Mouse GnRH neurons undergo dynamic remodeling in their morphology after birth, and this remodeling could have a functional significance [37]. During the pubertal transition, mouse GnRH neurons transform from having a complex dendritic tree bearing a few spines to having a simple dendritic structure bearing a large number of spines [37]. Consequently, the remodeled GnRH neurons in adults possess high dendritic spine densities, indicating the acquisition of abundant excitatory synaptic inputs [38] that could drive puberty. These observations contradict the previous reports that GnRH neurons receive sparse synaptic inputs [39, 40] and demonstrate pubertal onset is accompanied by the morphological maturation of GnRH neurons. Could FGF signaling be involved in the morphological maturation of postnatal GnRH neurons? Results from our laboratory suggest this is likely. We have shown that FGF signaling stimulates in vitro neurite branching of postnatal, but not embryonic, GnRH neurons [25]. Although the significance of this finding is unclear, it implicates FGF signaling in the postnatal alterations of GnRH neuronal morphology. Of further importance, dnFGFR female mice exhibit delayed puberty [20]. It stands to reason that delayed puberty in dnFGFR mice may be correlated with the reduced ability of their GnRH neurons to undergo morphological remodeling conducive to the receipt of excitatory inputs.

In addition to the postnatal maturation of GnRH neuronal morphology, FGF signaling could be required to maintain the postnatal GnRH system, thus promoting a healthy reproductive lifespan. Wu et al. [41] reported that there were ca. 1,100 GnRH neurons in neonatal mice, and this number declined to ca. 800 in adult mice. From then on, the number of GnRH neurons remained either unchanged [42] or declined only modestly by 18% in aging mice [43]. Overall, there does not appear to be a marked decrease in GnRH neurons with aging, suggesting GnRH neurons are unlikely to undergo dedifferentiation or cell death as they age. Rather, the aging GnRH system is more likely to undergo functional declines in GnRH synthesis and secretion [44]. Contrary to these observations, we show that postnatal dnFGFR mice, as they age, suffer a 70% loss in GnRH neurons and 95% loss in hypothalamic GnRH peptide concentration, respectively [26]. Our data suggest neurotrophic support by FGF signaling is absolutely critical for the maintenance of the postnatal GnRH system. In this sense, GnRH neurons are not unlike other neuronal systems such as motor neurons that rely heavily upon neurotrophic support for postnatal survival [45, 46]. Future studies are needed to examine the time course of postnatal GnRH neuronal loss and the mechanism underlying this loss.

Clinical Implications

Defective GnRH neuron migration was thought to be one of the major causes of IHH in all forms of KS. The lack of gross defects in GnRH neuronal migration in our dnFGFR, *Fgfr1* hypomorphic and *Fgf8* hypomorphic mice suggests that this extrapolation may not hold true for KS patients harboring loss-of-function mutations in *Fgfr1* and/or *Fgf8*. On the other hand, we have evidence indicating that disruption of FGFR1 and FGF8 signaling may have caused major defects during the fate specification phase of the GnRH system. Furthermore, our studies showed that FGF signaling is required for the postnatal maintenance and functionality of the GnRH neuronal system. Alltogether, a single mutated copy of the *Fgfr1* and/or *Fgf8* gene may lead to multiple insults on the GnRH neuronal system during prenatal and postnatal life.

Studies from mouse clearly showed that FGF signaling is involved, albeit not of equal importance, in all phases of GnRH neuronal development, maintenance, and functionality. For example, the global disruption of FGF signaling impacts primarily the fate specification phase of the GnRH neuronal system, whereas we did not observe gross abnormalities in GnRH neuronal migration. One might argue that if GnRH neurons were able to emerge, FGF signaling deficiency may still cause major migratory impairment later on. Our data from dnFGFR do not fully support this notion. In dnFGFR mice in which the tissue-specific disruption of FGFR occurs only after fate specification, GnRH neurons emerged normally, as expected (unpubl. data). After the emergence of these neurons, we observed only a slight arrest in GnRH neuronal migration [31]. The major GnRH system defect in these mice appears to be the precipitous postnatal loss of GnRH neurons that likely led to premature reproductive senescence. Based on these observations, we hypothesize that a heterozygous *Fgfr1* and/or *Fgf8* mutation in KS patients may lead to multiple insults on the GnRH neuronal system during fate specification and after birth. The postnatal loss of GnRH neurons may, in part, explain the manifestation of adult-onset IHH seen in a patient harboring *Fgf8* mutation [10].

Clinical observations showed that carrying a single identical gene mutation within and across IHH families is not predictive of the clinical reproductive and non-reproductive phenotypes, suggesting incomplete penetrance of a specific gene defect [47]. Another interesting and novel explanation for the lack of predictive precision could be that the severity of IHH depends on the number of gene defects found in a patient [47]. Indeed, Pitteloud et al. [47] identified a KS patient harboring heterozygous defects in both *Fgfr1* and *Nelf*. Recently, compound defects in *Fgfr1* and *Fgf8* have also been identified in two cases with normosmic IHH [10]. Although these invaluable clinical observations reveal the genetic complexity of IHH and KS, it is not possible to study directly in humans how these multiple mutations exacerbate IHH in KS patients. In theory, the mouse model could be extremely useful for testing the compound effects of such gene defects. For example, by crossbreeding *Fgfr1* hypomorphs with *Fgf8* hypomorphs, we can examine whether heterozygous defects on multiple IHH or KS-associated genes have compounding effects on the GnRH neuronal system.

KS patients represent a unique 'human model' that provides insights into signaling factors involved in the organization of a critical neuroendocrine system. Further elaboration on the molecular mechanisms induced by these factors is accomplished by studying transgenic mice. Using the mouse models, we have shown that FGF signaling is required not only for olfactory placode induction and differentiation, but also for fate specification and postnatal maintenance of the GnRH neuronal system. In sum, we speculate that IHH in KS is not merely a result of defective GnRH neuronal migration, but also insults accumulated in the GnRH system during pre- and postnatal development.

References

1 Schwanzel-Fukuda M, Pfaff DW: Origin of luteinizing hormone-releasing hormone neurons. Nature 1989;338:161–164.

2 Wray S, Grant P, Gainer H: Evidence that cells expressing luteinizing hormone-releasing hormone mRNA in the mouse are derived from progenitor cells in the olfactory placode. Proc Natl Acad Sci USA 1989;86:8132–8136.

3 Okubo K, Sakai F, Lau EL, Yoshizaki G, Takeuchi Y, Naruse K, Aida K, Nagahama Y: Forebrain gonadotropin-releasing hormone neuronal development: insights from transgenic medaka and the relevance to X-linked Kallmann syndrome. Endocrinology 2006;147:1076–1084.

4 Whitlock KE, Wolf CD, Boyce ML: Gonadotropin-releasing hormone (GnRH) cells arise from cranial neural crest and adenohypophyseal regions of the neural plate in the zebrafish, *Danio rerio*. Dev Biol 2003;257:140–152.

5 Schwanzel-Fukuda M: Origin and migration of luteinizing hormone-releasing hormone neurons in mammals. Microsc Res Tech 1999;44:2–10.

6 Tsai PS, Werner S, Weiner RI: Basic fibroblast growth factor is a neurotropic factor in GT1 gonadotropin-releasing hormone neuronal cell lines. Endocrinology 1995;136:3831–3838.

7 Dodé C, Levilliers J, Dupont JM, De Paepe A, Le Dû N, Soussi-Yanicostas N, Coimbra RS, Delmaghani S, Compain-Nouaille S, Baverel F, Pêcheux C, Le Tessier D, Cruaud C, Delpech M, Speleman F, Vermeulen S, Amalfitano A, Bachelot Y, Bouchard P, Cabrol S, Carel JC, Delemarre-van de Waal H, Goulet-Salmon B, Kottler ML, Richard O, Sanchez-Franco F, Saura R, Young J, Petit C, Hardelin JP: Loss-of-function mutations in FGFR1 cause autosomal dominant Kallmann syndrome. Nat Genet 2003;33:463–465.

8 Pitteloud N, Acierno JS Jr, Meysing A, Eliseenkova AV, Ma J, Ibrahimi OA, Metzger DL, Hayes FJ, Dwyer AA, Hughes VA, Yialamas M, Hall JE, Grant E, Mohammadi M, Crowley WF Jr: Mutations in fibroblast growth factor receptor 1 cause both Kallmann syndrome and normosmic idiopathic hypogonadotropic hypogonadism. Proc Natl Acad Sci USA 2006;103:6281–6286.

9 Pitteloud N, Meysing A, Quinton R, Acierno JS Jr, Dwyer AA, Plummer L, Fliers E, Boepple P, Hayes F, Seminara S, Hughes VA, Ma J, Bouloux P, Mohammadi M, Crowley WF Jr: Mutations in fibroblast growth factor receptor 1 cause Kallmann syndrome with a wide spectrum of reproductive phenotypes. Mol Cell Endocrinol 2006;254–255:60–69.

10 Falardeau J, Chung WCJ, Beenken A, Raivio T, Plummer L, Sidis Y, Jacobson-Dickman EE, Eliseenkova AV, Ma J, Dwyer AA, Quinton R, Na S, Hall JE, Huot C, Alois N, Pearce SH, Cole LW, Hughes VA, Mohammadi M, Tsai PS, Pitteloud N: Decreased FGF8 signaling causes deficiency of gonadotropin-releasing hormone in humans and mice. J Clin Invest 2008;118:2822–2831.

11 Ford-Perriss M, Abud H, Murphy M: Fibroblast growth factors in the developing central nervous system. Clin Exp Pharmacol Physiol 2001;28:493–503.

12 Wray S, Nieburgs A, Elkabes S: Spatiotemporal cell expression of luteinizing hormone-releasing hormone in the prenatal mouse: evidence for an embryonic origin in the olfactory placode. Brain Res Dev Brain Res 1989;46:309–318.

13 Wray S: Development of luteinizing hormone releasing hormone neurones. J Neuroendocrinol 2001;13:3–11.

14 Wray S, Key S, Qualls R, Fueshko SM: A subset of peripherin positive olfactory axons delineates the luteinizing hormone releasing hormone neuronal migratory pathway in developing mouse. Dev Biol 1994;166:349–354.

15 Livne I, Gibson MJ, Silverman AJ: Biochemical differentiation and intercellular interactions of migratory gonadotropin-releasing hormone (GnRH) cells in the mouse. Dev Biol 1993;159:643–656.

16 Merchenthaler I, Setalo G, Csontos C, Petrusz P, Flerko B, Negro-Vilar A: Combined retrograde tracing and immunocytochemical identification of luteinizing hormone-releasing hormone- and somatostatin-containing neurons projecting to the median eminence of the rat. Endocrinology 1989;125:2812–2821.

17 Silverman AJ, Silverman R, Lehman MN, Witkin JW, Millar RP: Localization of a peptide sequence contained in the precursor to gonadotropin releasing hormone (GnRH). Brain Res 1987;402:346–350.

18 Schwarting GA, Henion TR, Nugent JD, Caplan B, Tobet S: Stromal cell-derived factor-1 (chemokine C-X-C motif ligand 12) and chemokine C-X-C motif receptor 4 are required for migration of gonadotropin-releasing hormone neurons to the forebrain. J Neurosci 2006;26:6834–6840.
19 Tobet SA, Schwarting GA: Minireview: recent progress in gonadotropin-releasing hormone neuronal migration. Endocrinology 2006;147:1159–1165.
20 Tsai PS, Moenter SM, Postigo HR, El Majdoubi M, Pak TR, Gill JC, Paruthiyil S, Werner S, Weiner RI: Targeted expression of a dominant-negative fibroblast growth factor (FGF) receptor in gonadotropin-releasing hormone (GnRH) neurons reduces FGF responsiveness and the size of GnRH neuronal population. Mol Endocrinol 2005;19:225–236.
21 Partanen J, Schwartz L, Rossant J: Opposite phenotypes of hypomorphic and Y766 phosphorylation site mutations reveal a function for Fgfr1 in anteroposterior patterning of mouse embryos. Genes Dev 1998;12:2332–2344.
22 Colvin JS, Bohne BA, Harding GW, McEwen DG, Ornitz DM: Skeletal overgrowth and deafness in mice lacking fibroblast growth factor receptor 3. Nat Genet 1996;12:390–397.
23 Kawauchi S, Shou J, Santos R, Hébert JM, McConnell SK, Mason I, Calof A: Fgf8 expression defines a morphogenetic center required for olfactory neurogenesis and nasal cavity development in the mouse. Development 2005;132:5211–5223.
24 Itoh N, Ornitz DM: Evolution of the Fgf and Fgfr gene families. Trends Genet 2004;20:563–569.
25 Gill JC, Moenter SM, Tsai PS: Developmental regulation of gonadotropin-releasing hormone neurons by fibroblast growth factor signaling. Endocrinology 2004;145:3830–3839.
26 Chung WCJ, Moyle SS, Tsai PS: Fibroblast growth factor 8 signaling through Fgf receptor 1 is required for the emergence of gonadotropin-releasing hormone neurons. Endocrinology 2008;149:4997–5003.
27 Crossley PH, Martin GR: The mouse Fgf8 gene encodes a family of polypeptides and is expressed in regions that direct outgrowth and patterning in the developing embryo. Development 1995;121:439–451.
28 Meyers EN, Lewandoski M, Martin GR: An Fgf8 mutant allelic series generated by Cre- and Flp-mediated recombination. Nat Genet 1998;18:136–141.
29 Schwanzel-Fukuda M, Bick D, Pfaff DW: Luteinizing hormone-releasing hormone (LHRH)-expressing cells do not migrate normally in an inherited hypogonadal (Kallmann) syndrome. Brain Res Mol Brain Res 1989;6:311–326.
30 Schwanzel-Fukuda M, Crossin KL, Pfaff DW, Bouloux PM, Hardelin JP, Petit C: Migration of luteinizing hormone-releasing hormone (LHRH) neurons in early human embryos. J Comp Neurol 1996;366:547–557.
31 Tsai PS, Gill JC: Mechanisms of disease: insights into X-linked and autosomal-dominant Kallmann syndrome. Nat Clin Pract Endocrinol Metab 2006;2: 160–171.
32 Gill JC, Tsai PS: Expression of a dominant negative FGF receptor in developing GNRH1 neurons disrupts axon outgrowth and targeting to the median eminence. Biol Reprod 2006;74:463–472.
33 Silverman AJ, Zimmerman EA, Gibson MJ, Perlow MJ, Charlton HM, Kokoris GJ, Krieger DT: Implantation of normal fetal preoptic area into hypogonadal mutant mice: temporal relationships of the growth of gonadotropin-releasing hormone neurons and the development of the pituitary/testicular axis. Neuroscience 1985;16:69–84.
34 Rogers MC, Silverman AJ, Gibson MJ: Gonadotropin-releasing hormone axons target the median eminence: in vitro evidence for diffusible chemoattractive signals from the mediobasal hypothalamus. Endocrinology 1997;138:3956–3966.
35 Gibson MJ, Ingraham L, Dobrjansky A: Soluble factors guide gonadotropin-releasing hormone axonal targeting to the median eminence. Endocrinology 2000;141:3065–3071.
36 Hu Y, Guimond SE, Travers P, Cadman SM, Hohenester E, Turnbull JE, Kim SH, Bouloux PM: Novel mechanism of fibroblast growth factor receptor 1 regulation by extracellular matrix protein anosmin-1. J Biol Chem 2009;284:29905–29920.
37 Cottrell EC, Campbell RE, Han SK, Herbison AE: Postnatal remodeling of dendritic structure and spine density in gonadotropin-releasing hormone neurons. Endocrinology 2006;147:3652–3661.
38 Campbell RE, Han SK, Herbison AE: Biocytin filling of adult gonadotropin-releasing hormone neurons in situ reveals extensive, spiny, dendritic processes. Endocrinology 2005;146:1163–1169.
39 Witkin JW, O'Sullivan H, Silverman AJ: Novel associations among gonadotropin-releasing hormone neurons. Endocrinology 1995;136:4323–4330.
40 Witkin JW, Silverman AJ: Synaptology of luteinizing hormone-releasing hormone neurons in rat preoptic area. Peptides 1985;6:263–271.
41 Wu TJ, Gibson MJ, Rogers MC, Silverman AJ: New observations on the development of the gonadotropin-releasing hormone system in the mouse. J Neurobiol 1997;33:983–998.
42 Hoffman GE, Finch CE: LHRH neurons in the female C57BL/6J mouse brain during reproductive aging: no loss up to middle age. Neurobiol Aging 1986;7:45–48.

43 Miller MM, Joshi D, Billiar RB, Nelson JF: Loss of LH-RH neurons in the rostral forebrain of old female C57BL/6J mice. Neurobiol Aging 1990;11: 217–221.
44 Yin W, Gore AC: Neuroendocrine control of reproductive aging: roles of GnRH neurons. Reproduction 2006;131:403–414.
45 Holtmann B, Wiese S, Samsam M, Grohmann K, Pennica D, Martini R, Sendtner M: Triple knockout of CNTF, LIF, and CT-1 defines cooperative and distinct roles of these neurotrophic factors for motoneuron maintenance and function. J Neurosci 2005;25:1778–1787.
46 Sendtner M, Gotz R, Holtmann B, Escary JL, Masu Y, Carroll P, Wolf E, Brem G, Brulet P, Thoenen H: Cryptic physiological trophic support of motoneurons by LIF revealed by double gene targeting of CNTF and LIF. Curr Biol 1996;6:686–694.
47 Pitteloud N, Quinton R, Pearce SH, Raivio T, Acierno J, Dwyer AA, Plummer L, Hughes VA, Seminara SB, Cheng YZ, Li WP, Maccoll G, Eliseenkova AV, Olsen SK, Ibrahimi OA, Hayes FJ, Boepple P, Hall JE, Bouloux PM, Mohammadi M, Crowley WJ Jr: Digenic mutations account for variable phenotypes in idiopathic hypogonadotropic hypogonadism. J Clin Invest 2007;117:457–463.

Dr. Pei-San Tsai
Department of Integrative Physiology and Center for Neuroscience, University of Colorado at Boulder
114 Clare Small
Boulder, CO 80309-0354 (USA)
Tel. +1 303 735 1877, Fax +1 303 492 0811, E-Mail pei-san.tsai@colorado.edu

Quinton R (ed): Kallmann Syndrome and Hypogonadotropic Hypogonadism.
Front Horm Res. Basel, Karger, 2010, vol 39, pp 51–61

FGFR1 Mutations in Kallmann Syndrome

C. Villanueva · N. de Roux

Avenir Team 'Genetics and Physiology of Pubertal Onset', Inserm U676, Robert Debré Hospital, Paris Diderot University, Paris, France

Abstract

Kallmann syndrome (KS) is a heterogeneous genetic disorder that associates variable gonadotropin-releasing hormone (GnRH) deficiency with anosmia and, sometimes, other non-reproductive clinical features. X-linked recessive, as well as autosomal recessive and dominant modes of transmission have been described. The first KS-related gene to be described *(KAL1)* was in the X-linked form. The second gene *(KAL2)* was initially unexpected, as it was known to encode the fibroblast growth receptor 1 (FGFR1). Its consideration as a candidate gene arose as a result of cases with contiguous gene syndrome and, initially, mutations were mostly described in familial cases with autosomal dominant transmission of KS. Since its initial discovery, numerous mutations of *FGFR1* have been described in several functional domains of the receptor. Genotype-phenotype correlations have shown that some clinical features associated with KS, such as loss of nasal cartilage, hearing impairment, and anomalies of the limbs seem to be mainly associated with *KAL2* mutations. The role of FGFR1 in the normal development of the olfactory bulb explains the association of anosmia with GnRH deficiency in *FGFR1*-mutated patients. Phenotype analysis indicates that FGFR1 is involved in normal migration of GnRH fetal neurons, but this is clearly not the whole story as a substantial proportion of *KAL2*-mutated individuals have normosmic GnRH deficiency. Finally, recent additional observations, notably using animal models, but also the description of human mutations in a specific ligand of FGFR1, FGF8, are beginning to shed light on the pathogenesis of GnRH deficiency in general, not just KS.

Kallmann syndrome (KS) combines hypogonadotropic hypogonadism (HH) due to gonadotropin-releasing hormone (GnRH) deficiency and anosmia related to the absence or hypoplasia of the olfactory bulbs. KS is a genetically and clinically heterogeneous disorder that is 3–5 times more prevalent in males, in whom the prevalence is around 1 in 10,000 [1]. Many modes of inheritance have been described: X-linked, autosomal dominant and autosomal recessive. *KAL1* was identified by positional cloning strategies to underlie the X-chromosome-linked form of the disease, in which GnRH deficiency resulted from failed embryonic migration of GnRH-synthesizing neurons [2, 3]. Several reports have clearly demonstrated a direct link between loss of function of *KAL1* and KS phenotype. Non-reproductive features have also been reported, particularly mirror movements, renal aplasia, deafness and craniofacial and dental defects, although these are not consistent.

Despite the male-female excess of cases, autosomal dominant and recessive forms of KS are not explained by mutations in *KAL1*. The genetic causes of these autosomal familial forms were unexplained until the description of mutations within the gene encoding fibroblast growth factor receptor 1 *(FGFR1* or *KAL2)* in 2003 [4] and more recently, loss-of-function mutations in the gene encoding FGF8, which is one of FGFR1's natural ligands [5, 6]. Several reports then confirmed this initial description and indicated the very high clinical expressivity of KS due to *FGFR1* mutations. This unexpected result highlighted the role of FGFR1 in the normal development of the olfactory bulb in humans and especially its role in postnatal maturation of the gonadotropic axis.

FGFR1: An Unexpected Candidate Gene for Kallmann Syndrome

FGFR1 mutations were first described in a patient with a contiguous gene syndrome due to partial deletion of chromosome 8p. Three gene loci were present in the de novo 8p11.2-p12 deletion found in 2 affected individuals; from telomere to centromere, these genes were *WHSC1L1*, *FGFR1* and exons 1 and 2 of *TACCI* [4]. Dodé et al. [4] considered *FGFR1* to be the most interesting candidate gene as its invalidation results in olfactory bulb agenesis in mice and because it potentially interacts with the *KAL1* gene product anosmin-1. Several loss-of-function mutations were then described in other familial cases with autosomal transmission dominant transmission. This initial report was then confirmed by several groups [7].

FGFs and FGFRs play crucial roles, in vertebrate and invertebrate embryonic development, as growth factors that regulate cell proliferation, differentiation and migration. They are structurally related and they generally transmit extracellular signals to various cytoplasmic signal-transduction pathways through interaction with the extracellular domains of tyrosine kinase receptors. Indeed, mammalian FGF signaling begins at the cell surface through tightly regulated interactions of FGFR with FGFs, heparan sulfate proteoglycans, and other coreceptors [5] (fig. 1). Alternative splicing of *FGFR* transcripts generates a variety of FGFR isoforms with distinct FGF-binding specificities [8]. At least 11 ligands are able to activate FGFR1, and different functional domains have been described within its extracellular domain [9]. Two or three Ig-like domains, designated D1, D2, and D3, interfere with the binding affinity of FGFR1 toward FGF ligands. A stretch of acidic amino acids (acidic box domain AB) is located between Ig-like domains D1 and D2, followed by a heparin-binding region in D2. The C-terminal half of the D3 domain can be encoded by either exon 8a which determines the IIIb isoform or exon 8b, which encodes the IIIc isoform. The IIIb isoform is more highly expressed in epithelial

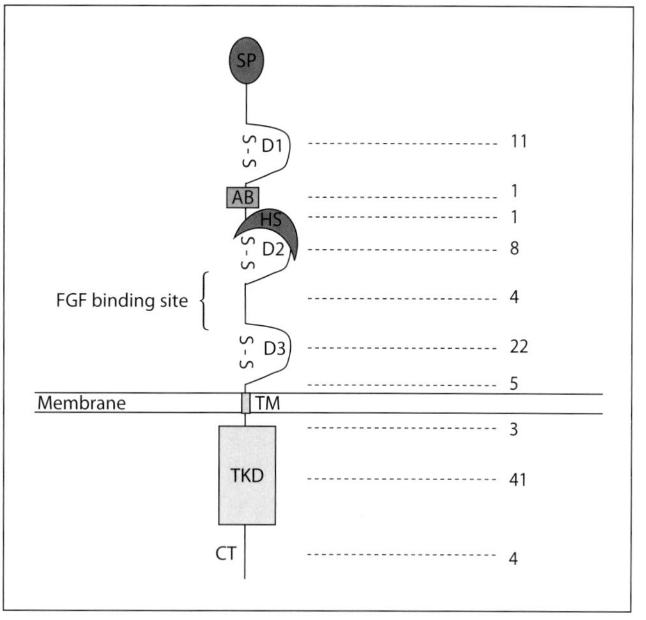

Fig. 1. Structure of FGFR1: signal peptide (SP), acidic box (AB), heparan sulphate binding site (HS), transmembrane domain (TM), TKD, immunoglobulin like domain D1, D2, D3, and C-terminal tail (CT). Number indicates mutation frequency (%) for each functional domain. Adapted from Kim et al. [7] and our unpublished mutations.

cells, the IIIc isoform in mesenchymal cells. The ligand binding site is located in the D2-D3 region. High-affinity FGF binding to the receptor requires heparan sulfate proteoglycan interaction with the extracellular domain. A soluble form of FGFR1, resulting from either proteolytic cleavage or secretion of the product of alternatively spliced mRNA transcript, has been described, but its biological role is unclear [10]. Both secreted and multiple proteolytically cleaved FGFRs are present in calf serum, but the relative contribution of each of these processes in vivo remains to be determined. FGF signal transduction during early embryonic development can proceed via three main intracellular pathways: Ras/MAP kinase, phospholipase C/calcium and PI3 kinase/Akt.

Mutations in *FGFR1*

While a single gain-of-function mutation in *FGFR1* (P252R) has been reported to cause a form of craniosynostosis [11], *FGFR1* mutations found in KS patients result in loss of function. Mutations of *FGFR1* have been described in the extracellular domain, the transmembrane domain, the intracellular domain and the tyrosine kinase domain (TKD). These mutations can be missense, nonsense, splice site or frameshift mutations, or intragenic insertions or deletions [12–22]. Some of them lead to more severe or less severe phenotypes and some others may be responsible for the 'reversible' phenotype. Some mutations affecting the D1 loop (R78C, V102I) may enhance the autoinhibitory state of FGFR1 [5]. Mutations in the D2 loop (Q237S, D224H and G237D) [14] or in the D3 loop (V273M, E274G, Y339C) destabilize the loop conformation, reducing the ligand-receptor interaction and most of the mutations described in the extracellular domain are found in the D3 loop (= 22% of the *FGFR1* mutations; fig. 1). Mutations were found in both major isoforms, FGFR1b and FGFR1c generated through alternative splicing in D3 loop indicating that FGFR1c, which is the minor form, is also involved in olfactory bulb development as well as palate morphogenesis [23]. Mutations in the intracellular domain reduce kinase activity and mutations in the TKD lead to a decrease in signal transduction [14]. For instance, both a nonsense mutation (Q680X) in the catalytic TKD of FGFR1 and a heterozygous double missense mutation (P772H and N724K) resulted in loss of function of FGFR1 by reducing tyrosine kinase activity [14]. The TKD mutations are the most frequently *FGFR1* described mutations (= 41%; fig. 1). Some mutations also occur in the acidic box and in the C-terminal tail [18]. All of these mutations result in congenitally deficient FGFR1 signaling, with variability in the observed phenotypes that will be discussed further.

The high phenotype specificity in humans due to FGFR1 inactivation was unexpected. In mice, invalidation of *FGFR1* leads to embryonic lethality at E9.5–E12 due to a more generalized cell migration defect, whereas targeted inactivation of *FGFR1* in the mouse telencephalon results in failure of olfactory bulb formation [24]. *FGFR1*-invalidated heterozygous mice do not have any phenotype [24]. Patients with heterozygous *FGFR1* deletions are very rare [7], though several nonsense mutations leading to premature STOP codon cause variable phenotypes (fig. 2). There is no experimental evidence of a potential dominant negative effect of mutated receptors on the wild-type receptor, suggesting that the phenotype results mainly from haploinsufficiency. This may explain why the phenotype due to *FGFR1*-inactivating mutations is so heterogeneous. It was therefore quite challenging to determine whether a specific FGFR1 ligand was involved in the normal development of the olfactory bulb. One could speculate that compensation should occur between each of the FGFR1 ligands. Again, the answer came from gene-invalidation studies in mice: transgenic mice hypomorphic for an *FGF8* allele exhibit olfactory bulb agenesis [25]. The role of FGF8 in the normal development of the olfactory bulb and, therefore, potentially also of normal migration of GnRH neurons in humans was recently demonstrated by Falardeau et al. [6], who described missense *FGF8* mutations in 6 cases of KS leading to various degrees of GnRH deficiency and olfactory phenotype.

Gonadotropic Axis Phenotype

Patients with *FGFR1* mutations show high variability in reproductive and non-reproductive phenotype; however, we have never observed a complete absence of

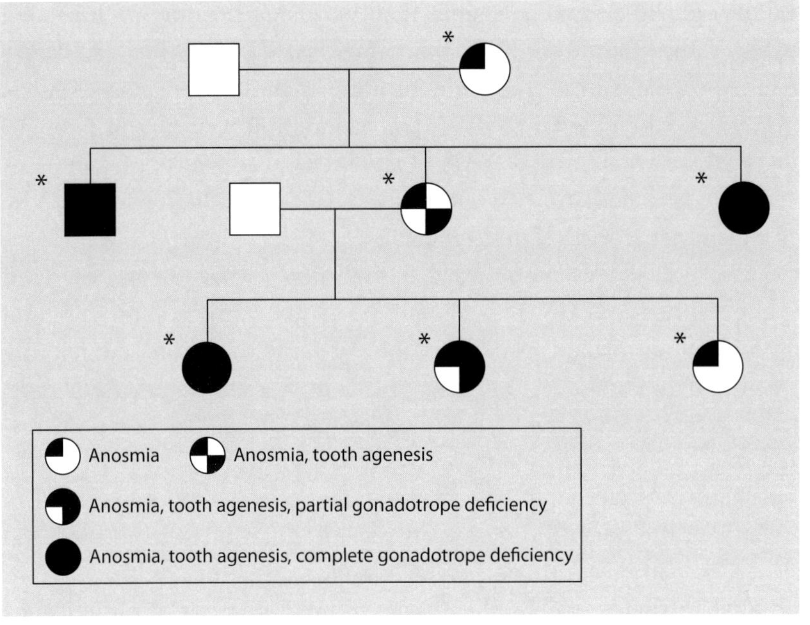

Fig. 2. Example of a high familial variability in the phenotype due to S139X mutation (*) in *FGFR1*. From Carel et al., unpubl. results.

clinical signs in patients bearing *FGFR1* loss-of-function mutations, nor has such an absence of signs ever convincingly been reported, to the best of our knowledge. In our strategy to screen for mutations, we first considered performing *FGFR1* sequencing in DNA extracted from patients with autosomal dominant or recessive forms of KS. Even if micropenis and cryptorchidism are the earliest clinical manifestations in *FGFR1*-mutated patients, in practice most present in adolescence with failed or arrested puberty, and a few adult cases are detected during workup for infertility.

We have clearly observed a slightly lesser degree of gonadotropic deficiency in patients with *FGFR1* mutations than in those with *KAL1* mutations, as recently reported by Salenave et al. [26]. This observation is not surprising as *KAL1* inactivation is expressed as a recessive trait without any discernible phenotype in women, whereas *FGFR1* mutations are mainly described as heterozygous mutations in both sexes. It is precisely this clinical heterogeneity, with partial gonadotropic deficiency in mutated patients, which has permitted the transmission of inactivating *FGFR1* mutations over generations. A few cases of compound heterozygotes or homozygotes have been reported in the familial form with recessive transmission [14, and our unpublished results]. Why some *FGFR1* mutations lead to dominant KS and others to the recessive form remains uncertain, but it does not seem to be related to the alteration in protein structure induced by the mutation.

The degree of hypogonadism and anosmia may vary significantly, even among siblings sharing the same mutations [14]: the same *FGFR1* mutation can cause hypogonadotropic hypogonadism with normal or abnormal olfaction. For instance, the mutation R622X described by Xu et al. [16] as a mutation resulting in hypogonadotropic hypogonadism with normal sense of smell has also been found in cases of hypogonadotropic hypogonadism with anosmia [4]. Reciprocally, anosmia can be combined with a wide range of GnRH deficiencies.

In contrast to the classical presentation of KS, few subjects have been described with reversible phenotype [19, 27]. Such a phenotype can be explained by impaired FGFR1 signaling and an abnormally small number of GnRH neurons completing their migration to the hypothalamus, resulting in incomplete pulse-generator maturation and partial hypogonadotropic hypogonadism [19]. This reversible phenotype was reported in a patient bearing a nonsense mutation in the TKD of FGFR1. The molecular mechanism underlying the reversible phenotype is unknown. It does not seem to be related to the type of mutation, as several mutations within the TKD have been described in patients with persistent hypogonadism in adulthood. Two hypotheses could explain the reversible phenotype. A small number of GnRH neurons appears to be sufficient for normal functioning of the gonadotropic axis [27]. The migration of GnRH neurons in these patients, previously thought to be completed during the fetal period, may continue in adulthood, increasing the number of GnRH neurons within the hypothalamus. One may also suspect a direct effect of testosterone on GnRH expression or maturation of synaptic projections to GnRH neurons. Androgen exposure is thus a potential modifier of the FGFR1 reproductive phenotype. The delayed puberty observed in transgenic mice expressing a dominant negative form of FGFR1 in the telencephalon demonstrated that FGFR1 signaling is required in the normal migration of GnRH neurons. These mice had a decreased population of GnRH neurons in the hypothalamus and a reduced number of GnRH axonal projections towards the median eminence. Cultured GnRH1 neurons expressing dominant negative FGFR1 exhibited attenuated activation of signaling pathways and reduced neurite outgrowth in response to FGF2, a ligand of FGFR1 in mice. These findings evidence a direct role for FGFR signaling in the guidance of GnRH1 axons to the median eminence [28]. The effect of FGF8 on the guidance of embryonic GnRH1 neurons needs to be tested to determine the relatedness of these mouse findings to human genetics.

KAL2 mutations account for about 10% of all cases of KS. Initially, Dodé et al. [4] described the prevalence for *FGFR1* mutations as 3% among familial cases and 6% among sporadic cases of KS in a Caucasian cohort, but other groups have subsequently observed significantly higher frequencies, e.g. Sato et al. [20] reporting prevalences of 11 and 9% of sporadic and familial cases, respectively, in a Japanese cohort, and Trarbach et al. [13] reporting a prevalence of 12% in a mixed population of 80 sporadic and familial idiopathic HH (IHH) cases. Zenaty et al. [21] described pediatric cases with *FGFR1* mutations, showing that de novo mutations are infrequent and that the severity of orofacial malformation at birth does not predict gonadotropic function at normal age of pubertal onset.

The genetic basis of many sporadic cases of both normosmic IHH and KS (which represent the majority of patients) remains unknown, as does the reason for the excess of male cases. Recently, Pitteloud et al. [22] proposed that two different gene defects can synergize to produce a more severe phenotype than either defect alone. For instance, a proband carrying a heterozygous mutation in both *FGFR1* and *NELF* (nasal embryonic LHRH factor) genes exhibited a more severe KS phenotype, with cleft palate, than other siblings carrying either the *FGFR1* or *NELF* mutation alone. Similarly, a heterozygotic mutation of *FGFR1* was described in a pair of sisters also bearing two compound heterozygotic mutations of the GnRH receptor gene *(GnRHR)* [22]. A more pronounced phenotype was described in these 2 females than in an unrelated patient bearing the same GnRHR compound heterozygotic mutations [29]. Although more cases are emerging, e.g. Canto et al. [30], the frequency of these digenic or oligogenic cases remains thus far insufficient to explain the high frequency of sporadic KS and normosmic IHH.

Non-Reproductive Phenotypes

Recent investigations of loss-of-function *FGFR1* mutations have been performed to clarify the role of this growth factor in the clinical signs associated with hypogonadism and anosmia in KS. Apart from anosmia, a variety of phenotypic anomalies may be observed alongside IHH, occasionally resulting from a contiguous gene syndrome, e.g. red blood cell spherocytosis due to codeletion of both ankyrin and *FGFR1* genes at 8p11-p12 [4]. More typically, studies of *KAL2* human mutations and of mutant *FGFR1*-invalidated mice have shown a high prevalence of cleft lip and/or palate, consistent with the role of FGF signaling in palate formation.

FGFR1 is ubiquitously expressed during brain development with high levels of expression reported in the forebrain and midbrain. FGFR1 and FGFR2 are broadly expressed in facial mesenchyme and ectoderm, respectively [31]. FGFR1 patterns the pharyngeal region to create a permissive environment for neural crest migration [32]. Mice homozygous for hypomorphic alleles of *FGFR1* die neonatally and have craniofacial defects. Eighty percent of these *FGFR1* mutants have open palate shelves, and variable deficiency has been observed in their middle ear ossicles [32]. The neural crest of the second arch of these mutants initially forms normally and migrates ventrally, but then fails to enter the second branchial arch. Humans with *FGFR1* mutations also show cleft lip and/or palate in 25–30% of cases [17]. This clinical feature is also present (though at much lower frequency) in *KAL1* patients, who may also show a more high-arched palate [17]. Other clinical features have only been reported in *FGFR1/KAL2* patients, such as loss of nasal cartilage, hypo- or aplasia of the external ear with hearing impairment, anomalies of the limb, and tooth agenesis [17].

Hypogonadism in KS has been classified as a form of IHH caused by defects in GnRH neuron development due to multigenic etiology, with modifier genes influencing the phenotypic outcome. FGFR1 expression has been detected in the nasal placode, developing olfactory bulb, GnRH migratory pathways, GnRH neurons and their projections. Mutant mice that do not express FGFR1 in the telencephalon show normal initial contact between olfactory axons and the forebrain, but the olfactory bulb does not evaginate from the neuroepithelial wall [24]. A large proportion of the neuroepithelial cells in the rostral forebrain continue dividing, whereas normal mice show a local decrease in cell proliferation before olfactory bulb evagination. The mutant mice die shortly after birth because of their inability to suck resulting from their smelling impairment. One important FGFR1 ligand, FGF8, is detected in olfactory epithelium neuronal cell lineages, and its inactivation in mice leads to the absence of an olfactory bulb and midline defects [25]. These data demonstrate that FGFR1 is required in normal midbrain and craniofacial development.

Anosmin, which is encoded by *KAL1*, may be one of the key factors in determining the outcome of FGFR1 signaling leading to neuronal differentiation and migration [7]. Normal FGFR1 signaling is required for normal number and migration of GnRH neurons before birth. It may play a role in the organization of the central terminal nerve roots, which normally guide the GnRH neurons as they penetrate into the forebrain [33]. However, FGF signaling could be important in the migration process as well [34]. Anosmin-1, responsible for the X-linked form of KS, is indeed involved in axon branching and may interact with FGFR1 [35]. Anosmin binds to the extracellular domain of FGFR1 via a heparan sulfate-dependent pathway [7]. This interaction facilitates the ligand-receptor interaction regulating FGFR1 intracellular pathways by increasing the duration and intensity of FGFR1 activation via MAPK phosphorylation [36, 37]. This MAPK pathway has been implicated in neurite outgrowth in different neuronal cell lines via changes in the cytoskeleton [7]. The hypothesis that anosmin-1 also modulates the binding of FGF8 to FGFR1 remains to be tested.

Conclusions

FGFR1 plays a pivotal role in KS pathogenesis and an essential role during early stages of development. Analysis of *FGFR1* mutant mice and especially of conditional *FGFR1* mice has provided valuable information on the role of this receptor in olfactory bulb morphogenesis and GnRH neuron ontogeny. Moreover, these conditional mice have provided an explanation for some of the clinical features associated with hypogonadotropic hypogonadism in KS, such as limb anomalies, cleft palate and dental agenesis.

Analysis of human phenotypes related to *FGFR1* mutations has provided similar important information. A wide spectrum of reproductive phenotypes in KS subjects carrying *FGFR1* mutations is observed. This variability indicates that, at least in some patients, any defect in GnRH migration is not absolute. The variability of phenotypes among family members carrying the same mutation also suggests important interactions of *FGFR1* with other modifier genes. Functional interactions between proteins encoded by these genes and the relative roles of each in the pathogenesis of KS need to be further specified.

References

1 Hu Y, Tanriverdi F, MacColl GS, Bouloux PM: Kallmann's syndrome: molecular pathogenesis. Int J Biochem Cell Biol 2003;35:1157–1162.

2 Franco B, Guioli S, Pragliola A, Incerti B, Bardoni B, Tonlorenzi R, Carrozzo R, Maestrini E, Pieretti M, Taillon-Miller P, Brown CJ, Willard HF, Lawrence C, Persico MG, Camerino G, Ballabio A: A gene deleted in Kallmann's syndrome shares homology with neural cell adhesion and axonal path-finding molecules. Nature 1991;353:529–536.

3 Legouis R, Hardelin JP, Levilliers J, Claverie JM, Compain S, Wunderle V, Millasseau P, Le Paslier D, Cohen D, Caterina D, Bouguerelet L, Delemarre-Van de Waal, Lutfalla G, Wessenbach J, Petit C: The candidate gene for the X-linked Kallmann syndrome encodes a protein related to adhesion molecules. Cell 1991;67:423–435.

4 Dodé C, Levilliers J, Dupont JM, De Paepe A, Le Dû N, Soussi-Yanicostas N, Coimbra RS, Delmaghani S, Compain-Nouaille S, Baverel F, Pêcheux C, Le Tessier D, Cruaud C, Delpech M, Speleman F, Vermeulen S, Amalfitano A, Bachelot Y, Bouchard P, Cabrol S, Carel JC, Delemarre-van de Waal H, Goulet-Salmon B, Kottler ML, Richard O, Sanchez-Franco F, Saura R, Young J, Petit C, Hardelin JP: Loss-of-function mutations in FGFR1 cause autosomal dominant Kallmann syndrome. Nat Genet 2003;33:463–465.

5 Mohammadi M, Olsen SK, Ibrahimi OA: Structural basis for fibroblast growth factor receptor activation. Cytokine Growth Factor Rev 2005;16:107–137.

6 Falardeau J, Chung WC, Beenken A, Raivio T, Plummer L, Sidis Y, Jacobson-Dickman EE, Eliseenkova AV, Ma J, Dwyer AA, Quinton R, Na S, Hall JE, Huot C, Alois N, Pearce SH, Cole LW, Hughes V, Mohammadi M, Tsai PS, Pitteloud N: Decreased FGF8 signaling causes deficiency of gonadotropin-releasing hormone in humans and mice. J Clin Invest 2008;118:2822–2831.

7 Kim SH, Hu Y, Cadman S, Bouloux P: Diversity in fibroblast growth factor receptor 1 regulation: learning from the investigation of Kallmann syndrome. J Neuroendocrinol 2008;20:141–163.

8 Böttcher RT, Niehrs C: Fibroblast growth factor signaling during early vertebrate development. Endocr Rev 2005;26:63–77.

9 Zhang X, Ibrahimi OA, Olsen SK, Umemori H, Mohammadi M, Ornitz DM: Receptor specificity of the fibroblast growth factor family. The complete mammalian FGF family. J Biol Chem 2006;281: 15694–15700.

10 Hanneken A: Structural characterization of the circulating soluble FGF receptors reveals multiple isoforms generated by secretion and ectodomain shedding. FEBS Lett 2001;489:176–181.

11 Muenke M, Schell U, Hehr A, Robin NH, Losken HW, Schinzel A, Pulleyn LJ, Rutland P, Reardon W, Malcolm S, Winter RM: A common mutation in the fibroblast growth factor receptor 1 gene in Pfeiffer syndrome. Nat Genet 1994;8:269–274.

12 Sato N, Hasegawa T, Hori N, Fukami M, Yoshimura Y, Ogata T: Gonadotrophin therapy in Kallmann syndrome caused by heterozygous mutations of the gene for fibroblast growth factor receptor 1: report of three families: case report. Hum Reprod 2005;20: 2173–2178.

13 Trarbach EB, Costa EM, Versiani B, de Castro M, Baptista MT, Garmes HM, de Mendonca BB, Latronico AC: Novel fibroblast growth factor receptor 1 mutations in patients with congenital hypogonadotropic hypogonadism with and without anosmia. J Clin Endocrinol Metab 2006;91:4006–4012.

14 Pitteloud N, Acierno JS Jr, Meysing A, Eliseenkova AV, Ma J, Ibrahimi OA, Metzger DL, Hayes FJ, Dwyer AA, Hughes VA, Yialamas M, Hall JE, Grant E, Mohammadi M, Crowley WF Jr: Mutations in fibroblast growth factor receptor 1 cause both Kallmann syndrome and normosmic idiopathic hypogonadotropic hypogonadism. Proc Natl Acad Sci USA 2006;103:6281–6286.

15 Pedersen-White JR, Chorich LP, Bick DP, Sherins RJ, Layman LC: The prevalence of intragenic deletions in patients with idiopathic hypogonadotropic hypogonadism and Kallmann syndrome. Mol Hum Reprod 2008;14:367–370.

16 Xu N, Qin Y, Reindollar RH, Tho SP, McDonough PG, Layman LC: A mutation in the fibroblast growth factor receptor 1 gene causes fully penetrant normosmic isolated hypogonadotropic hypogonadism. J Clin Endocrinol Metab 2007;92:1155–1158.

17 Hardelin JP, Dodé C: Kallmann syndrome. Eur J Hum Genet 2009;17:138–146.

18 Albuisson J, Pêcheux C, Carel JC, Lacombe D, Leheup B, Lapuzina P, Bouchard P, Legius E, Matthijs G, Wasniewska M, Delpech M, Young J, Hardelin JP, Dodé C: Kallmann syndrome: 14 novel mutations in KAL1 and FGFR1 (KAL2). Hum Mutat 2005;25:98–99.

19 Pitteloud N, Acierno JS Jr, Meysing AU, Dwyer AA, Hayes FJ, Crowley WF Jr: Reversible Kallmann syndrome, delayed puberty, and isolated anosmia occurring in a single family with a mutation in the fibroblast growth factor receptor 1 gene. J Clin Endocrinol Metab 2005;90:1317–1322.

20 Sato N, Katsumata N, Kagami M, Hasegawa T, Hori N, Kawakita S, Minowada S, Shimotsuka A, Shishiba Y, Yokozawa M, Yasuda T, Nagasaki K, Hasegawa D, Hasegawa Y, Tachibana K, Naiki Y, Horikawa R, Tanaka T, Ogata T: Clinical assessment and mutation analysis of Kallmann syndrome 1 (KAL1) and fibroblast growth factor receptor 1 (FGFR1, or KAL2) in five families and 18 sporadic patients. J Clin Endocrinol Metab 2004;89:1079–1088.

21 Zenaty D, Bretones P, Lambe C, Guemas I, David M, Leger J, de Roux N: Paediatric phenotype of Kallmann syndrome due to mutations of fibroblast growth factor receptor 1 (FGFR1). Mol Cell Endocrinol 2006;254–255:78–83.

22 Pitteloud N, Quinton R, Pearce SH, Raivio T, Acierno J, Dwyer AA, Plummer L, Hughes VA, Seminara SB, Cheng YZ, Li WP, MacColl GS, Eliseenkova AV, Olsen SK, Ibrahimi OA, Hayes FJ, Boepple P, Hall JE, Bouloux PM, Mohammadi M, Crowley W: Digenic mutations account for variable phenotypes in idiopathic hypogonadotropic hypogonadism. J Clin Invest 2007;117:457–463.

23 Dodé C, Fouveaut C, Mortier G, Janssens S, Bertherat J, Mahoudeau J, Kottler ML, Chabrolle C, Gancel A, François I, Devriendt K, Wolczynski S, Pugeat M, Pineiro-Garcia A, Murat A, Bouchard P, Young J, Delpech M, Hardelin JP: Novel FGFR1 sequence variants in Kallmann syndrome, and genetic evidence that the FGFR1c isoform is required in olfactory bulb and palate morphogenesis. Hum Mutat 2007;28:97–98.

24 Hébert JM, Lin M, Partanen J, Rossant J, McConnell SK: FGF signaling through FGFR1 is required for olfactory bulb morphogenesis. Development 2003;130:1101–1111.

25 Meyers EN, Lewandoski M, Martin GR: An Fgf8 mutant allelic series generated by Cre- and Flp-mediated recombination. Nat Genet 1998;18:136–141.

26 Salenave S, Chanson P, Bry H, Pugeat M, Cabrol S, Carel JC, Murat A, Lecomte P, Brailly S, Hardelin JP, Dodé C, Young J: Kallmann's syndrome: a comparison of the reproductive phenotypes in men carrying KAL1 and FGFR1/KAL2 mutations. J Clin Endocrinol Metab 2008;93:758–763.

27 Ribeiro RS, Vieira TC, Abucham J: Reversible Kallmann syndrome: report of the first case with a KAL1 mutation and literature review. Eur J Endocrinol 2007;156:285–290.

28 Gill JC, Tsai PS: Expression of a dominant negative FGF receptor in developing GNRH1 neurons disrupts axon outgrowth and targeting to the median eminence. Biol Reprod 2006;74:463–472.

29 de Roux N, Young J, Misrahi M, Genet R, Chanson P, Schaison G, Milgrom E: A family with hypogonadotropic hypogonadism and mutations in the gonadotropin-releasing hormone receptor. N Engl J Med 1997;337:1597–1602.

30 Canto P, Munguía P, Söderlund D, Castro JJ, Méndez JP: Genetic analysis in patients with Kallmann syndrome: coexistence of mutations in prokineticin receptor 2 and KAL1. J Androl 2009;30:41–45.

31 Bachler M, Neubüser A: Expression of members of the Fgf family and their receptors during midfacial development. Mech Dev 2001;100:313–316.

32 Trokovic N, Trokovic R, Mai P, Partanen J: Fgfr1 regulates patterning of the pharyngeal region. Genes Dev 2003;17:141–153.

33 Dodé C, Hardelin JP: Kallmann syndrome: fibroblast growth factor signaling insufficiency? J Mol Med 2004;82:725–734.

34 Gill JC, Moenter SM, Tsai PS: Developmental regulation of gonadotropin-releasing hormone neurons by fibroblast growth factor signaling. Endocrinology 2004;145:3830–3839.

35 Soussi-Yanicostas N, de Castro F, Julliard AK, Perfettini I, Chédotal A, Petit C: Anosmin-1, defective in the X-linked form of Kallmann syndrome, promotes axonal branch formation from olfactory bulb output neurons. Cell 2002;109:217–228.
36 Hu Y, Guimond SE, Travers P, Cadman SM, Hohenester E, Turnbull JE, Kim SH, Bouloux PM: Novel mechanism of fibroblast growth factor receptor 1 regulation by extracellular matrix protein anosmin-1. J Biol Chem 2009;284:29905–29920.
37 González-Martínez D, Kim SH, Hu Y, Guimond S, Schofield J, Winyard P, Vannelli GB, Turnbull J, Bouloux PM: Anosmin-1 modulates fibroblast growth factor receptor 1 signaling in human gonadotropin-releasing hormone olfactory neuroblasts through a heparan sulfate-dependent mechanism. J Neurosci 2004;24:10384–10392.

Nicolas de Roux, MD, PhD
Avenir team 'Genetics and Physiology of Pubertal Onset'
Inserm U676, Robert Debré Hospital, Paris Diderot University
48 Bd Sérurier, FR–75019 Paris (France)
Tel. +33 1 40 03 19 85, Fax +33 1 40 03 19 95, E-Mail nicolas.deroux@inserm.fr

Quinton R (ed): Kallmann Syndrome and Hypogonadotropic Hypogonadism.
Front Horm Res. Basel, Karger, 2010, vol 39, pp 62–77

Biology of *KAL1* and Its Orthologs: Implications for X-Linked Kallmann Syndrome and the Search for Novel Candidate Genes

Gavin S. MacColl[a] · Richard Quinton[a] · Hannes E. Bülow[b]

[a]Endocrine Research Group, Institute of Human Genetics, University of Newcastle-upon-Tyne, Newcastle-upon-Tyne, UK; [b]Department of Genetics and Dominick P. Purpura Department of Neuroscience, Albert Einstein College of Medicine, New York, N.Y., USA

Abstract

Kallmann syndrome is characterised by congenital hypogonadotropic hypogonadism and anosmia, sometimes with other non-reproductive defects. Although multiple genetic pathways are now known to be involved in the development of this disorder, *KAL1*, the gene causing the X-linked form of Kallmann syndrome was the first to be identified. It has thus been extensively studied both in vitro and in vivo, though the absence of an identifiable murine ortholog has denied researchers the opportunity to create and study *Kal-1* knock-out mice. This review looks at several studies in species with a *kal-1* ortholog, revealing functional similarities with the human disorder. Further work has shown that the *kal-1* domain structure is maintained across genera, that it controls similar morphological and cellular processes during development, and that data from the nematode *Caenorhabditis elegans*, in particular, may point to novel human candidate genes.

Kallmann Syndrome Phenotypes and Definitions

Kallmann syndrome (KS) is defined by isolated (or idiopathic) hypogonadotropic hypogonadism (IHH) and anosmia. These olfactory and reproductive deficits are combined with a variable non-reproductive phenotype, including cryptorchidism, bimanual synkinesis (mirror movements), renal agenesis, craniofacial or dental abnormalities, syndactyly, coloboma and sensorineural deafness [1–3]. In 1991, two groups that had been working independently published their positional cloning data identifying the gene that came to be known as *KAL1* [4, 5]. Not long before, the neuroanatomic examination of a single 19-week human fetus bearing an Xpter deletion that encompassed the *KAL1* locus had suggested that low or absent LH pulses in adult life in X-linked KS (X-KS) were the result of an embryonic GnRH-1 neuron migratory defect [6]. Despite the male preponderance of IHH cases, which might suggest the predominance of the X-linked mode of inheritance, in fact less than 10% of unrelated IHH males in the Harvard/Massachusetts General Hospital patient series harbour *KAL1* coding sequence mutations (Pitteloud, pers. commun.).

It has since been established that X-KS males seem to have a particularly severe neuroendocrine phenotype, with severe androgen deficiency characterised by complete LH apulsatility and azoospermia, a higher prevalence of childhood cryptorchism and near-100% association between anosmia and IHH among affected individuals [2, 3, 7]. Moreover instances of non-classical disease, e.g. adult-onset IHH, KS-with-reversal, or incomplete penetrance in males harbouring *KAL1* coding sequence mutations are conspicuous by their rarity [8, 9]. Anosmia results from agenesis or dysgenesis of the olfactory bulbs and secondary processing regions [1, 6, 10, 11]. Mirror movements (bimanual synkinesis) and unilateral renal agenesis are both characteristic of, though not exclusive to X-KS. The former seem to result from an abnormally hypertrophic ipsilateral corticospinal tract, as shown by a combination of electrophysiological, functional positron emission tomography and MRI morphometry studies [12–15].

KAL-1 and X-Linked Kallmann Syndrome

KAL1, a Human Gene with No Rodent Ortholog

The X-linked form of KS (X-KS) is caused by mutations in *KAL-1*, located at Xp22.3. *KAL-1* has 14 exons and encodes anosmin-1, an extracellular matrix protein with a modular structure consisting of a cysteine rich region, a whey acidic protein (WAP) domain, four fibronectin type III (FnIII) domains and a histidine-rich region. Many of the mutations in *KAL-1* that cause X-KS affect the WAP and FnIII domains, either leading to truncated forms of the anosmin-1 protein through creation of premature STOP codons, or substitution of key amino acids that are essential for its various biological functions. These point mutations have been modelled in vitro [5, 16–19]. Several of these mutations in *KAL-1*, the corresponding amino acid substitutions, and their biological phenotype and characterisation, are shown in table 1.

The *KAL-1* gene has orthologous and paralogous sequences in diverse animal genera and species, a small number of which are genetically tractable allowing modelling of function in vivo [20–22]. However, despite the impressive neuroanatomical links between olfactory, pheromonal and GnRH-1 neuron development seen in rodents, reflecting the profound interactions that mediate their social and reproductive behaviours, there does not appear to be a rodent *Kal-1* ortholog [23–25]. Nevertheless, several rodent models have been used to study GnRH-1 neuron development in vivo under the influence of a variety of different genetic backgrounds (table 2).

Table 1. Examples of phenotypes associated with *KAL-1* mutations

KAL-1 mutation	Domain(s) affected	Phenotype(s)	Study
E514K	FnIII-3	anosmia, IHH, unilateral renal agenesis	[59, 60]
N267K	FnIII-1	anosmia, IHH, bimanual synkinesis, unilateral renal agenesis	[16]
C172R	WAP	anosmia, IHH, LH apulsatility, bimanual synkinesis	[61]
R191X	Exon 5	bimanual synkinesis, unilateral renal agenesis	[62]

Table 2. Altered GnRH-1 neuron migration pathways in rodents

Gene affected	GnRH-1 neuron migration defect?	Phenotype	Study
EphrinA5	yes	arrested GnRH-1 cell clusters in the olfactory region	[63]
Dcc/Netrin	yes	misrouting of GnRH-1 neurons to the cortex	[64, 65]
Fgf8	yes	elimination/lack of emergence of GnRH-1 neurons; no vomeronasal organ	[66]
Fgfr1	yes	reduced GnRH-1 cell numbers in the preoptic area of FGFR1 hypomorphs	[66]

GnRH-1 Neuron Migratory Route

GnRH-1 neurons follow a complex route through the developing olfactory system, originating in the medial olfactory placode, and migrating into the forebrain and eventually to the hypothalamus [6, 23, 24]. The migratory pathway of GnRH-1 neurons may be divided into several stages including neurogenesis and exit from the medial olfactory placode, migration into the forebrain, and differentiation into neurosecretory cells that release GnRH-1 into the circulation [26, 27].

How do mutations in *KAL-1* influence the migratory behaviour of GnRH-1 cells? The single histological study of a 19-week human fetus harbouring an Xpter deletion evidenced that deletion of *KAL1* resulted in GnRH-1 neurons becoming trapped in the upper nasal region, with absent GnRH-1 immunoreactivity within the CNS. Axons of the olfactory, terminal and vomeronasal nerves (the cranial nerve I complex) failed to establish synaptic contacts within the forebrain, instead ending in neural tangles underneath the meninges overlying the cribriform plate; the olfactory bulbs were absent [6].

KAL-1 and Olfactory Development

KAL-1 is expressed in the mitral and glomerular layers of the developing olfactory bulbs; anosmin-1 also envelopes the extracellular matrices of the developing

Table 3. *Kal-1* domain structure in selected species

Species	Domains	Expression pattern	Studies
D. melanogaster	WAP/2×FnIII	gonadal precursors, head region	[20, 37]
O. latipes	WAP/4×FnIII	olfactory bulb, medial telencephalon, branchial arches, cerebellum, pectoral fin	[20]
C. elegans	WAP/4×FnIII	larval and adult neurons in several head ganglia, labial sensory neurons, motor neurons in the ventral nerve cord	[20]
G. gallus	WAP/4×FnIII	developing olfactory bulbs	[32]
M. mulatta	WAP/4×FnIII	no data	

telencephalon – supporting a role for *KAL-1* in the development of the early olfactory regions [28, 29]. Incubation of rodent olfactory bulb explants with cells stably expressing the *KAL-1* cDNA also stimulates neurite outgrowth from tissue explants [10].

Kal-1 Orthologs in Other Species

Many species have orthologous Kal-1 genes, whose predicted protein domain organisation shares structural similarities with the human form [30], thereby allowing modelling of domain function in vivo. Species where in vivo *kal-1* expression and function have been studied in detail include *Gallus gallus*, and the genetically more tractable organisms *Danio rerio*, *Caenorhabditis elegans* and *Drosophila melanogaster* (table 3). Due to a whole genome duplication event occurring in the ray-fin fish lineage, zebrafish and medaka have two *KAL1* orthologs known as *kal-1a* (or *kal1.1*) encoding anosmin-1a and *kal-1b* (or *kal-1.2*) encoding anosmin-1b. A phylogenetic tree of the vertebrate *Kal-1* family, using *C. elegans* as outroot, shows that this gene duplication predated the emergence of teleosts and tetrapods, and that *kal-1.1* is orthologous to *KAL1*, whereas *kal-1.2* is paralogous (fig. 1). Based on their non-overlapping expression patterns, these two genes are considered to have separate roles [22, 31].

Avian kal

The chick *kal-1* gene is expressed in multiple neuronal sites during development, shown by in situ hybridization using primer oligonucleotides against exon III, which shares up to 89% sequence homology with human *KAL1* [32]. Between embryonic day 6 (E6) and E8, the chick *Kal* transcript is present in the germinal layer of the developing neural tube. From E8 onwards, it is present in the developing olfactory

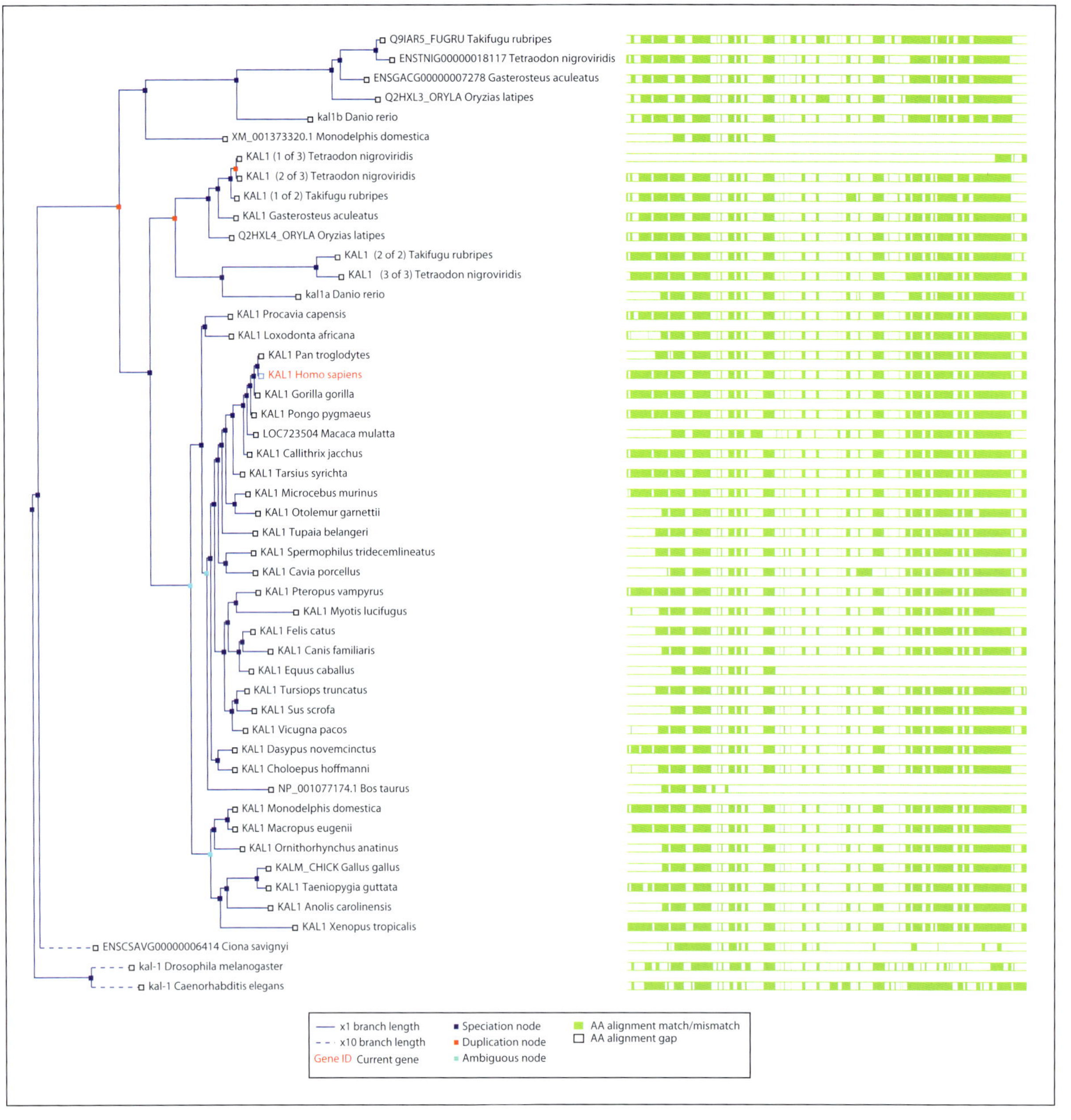

Fig. 1. Phylogenetic tree for *Homo sapiens KAL1*. Adapted from Ensembl.

bulb, particularly in the mitral cell layer, and also in cerebellar purkinje cells, retinal neurons and some neuron populations in the brainstem and spinal cord. At later stages transcription in olfactory bulb mitral cells became more intense, with a few olfactory bulb tufted cells also expressing *Kal*. This expression pattern decreases in intensity from E16 onwards. In contrast, low levels or absent expression are observed in the developing kidney, olfactory epithelium and the surrounding nasal mesenchyme [32, 33].

Zebrafish kal Genes

The study of *Kal-1* function in vertebrates was initially held back by the lack of a genetically tractable mammalian model to study the effects of orthologous sequences on GnRH-1 neuron development. However, two recent studies demonstrating similar functionality of *Kal-1* orthologs in chordate fish have established anosmin-1 as having an essential and evolutionarily conserved role during GnRH neuronal migration from the nasal area into the brain [21, 22]. In zebrafish, a sequence comparison between human *KAL1* and the zebrafish *kal-1.1/1.2* orthologs demonstrated 68% similarity at the level of protein sequence and a high degree of sequence similarity between the WAP and FnIII domains from both species [31].

In situ hybridisation shows transcription of *kal-1.1* and *kal-1.2* genes in various neuronal structures; at embryonic stage 38 h.p.f, *kal-1.1* transcript is produced in the presumptive olfactory bulbs (though not in the adult olfactory system) and, at lower levels, in other embryonic tissues including the midbrain, tectum, cerebellum, retina and spinal cord [31]. It is also expressed in sensory hair cells of the inner ear and lateral line, evidencing a role in ear development [34]. The *kal-1.2* transcript is present at lower levels at stage 48 h.p.f. onwards in the epithelium of the nasal cavity, the rostral telencephalic area, the cerebral lobes and the pronephric duct [31].

Effect of kal-1.1 Knockdown on Hypothalamic GnRH Cells in Zebrafish

Does a loss of function of *kal-1.1* and *kal-1.2* genes affect GnRH-1 cell numbers in the zebrafish hypothalamus? Morpholino knockdown of *kal-1.1* translation completely eliminated the hypothalamic GnRH-1 cell population, without affecting the development of midbrain GnRH-2, or terminal nerve GnRH-3 cells, supporting a specific role for *kal-1.1* in the development of the endocrine GnRH-1 system in zebrafish. By contrast, a similar knockdown of *kal-1.2* resulted in only a slight reduction in the number of hypothalamic GnRH-1 neurons and, again, no effect on GnRH-2 and GnRH-3 neuron populations. Thus, in zebrafish, *kal-1.2* plays the dominant role in migration and development of endocrine GnRH cells, but development of the GnRH-2 and GnRH-3 systems (whose roles are neuromodulatory rather than endocrine) must therefore be regulated via separate pathways [21].

Interestingly, knockdown of *kal-1.1*, but not *kal-1.2*, severely impaired posterior lateral line primordium (PLLP) migration [35]. The lateral line is a mechanosensory organ, comprising rows of neuromasts containing sensory hair cells and phylogenetically related to the inner ear of land vertebrates that allows fish to sense water movements and avoid obstacles. The PLLP originates from a sensory placode and migrates towards the tail, whilst also undergoing a process of differentiation. The PLLP was shown to express high levels of both *kal-1.1* and *kal-1.2*. Further, *Kal-1.1* morpholinos disrupted PLLP migration, although neuromast differentiation within the PLLP was not impaired [35].

Kal Knockdown in Medaka

Medaka *(Oryzias latipes)* also has two orthologous sequences, *kal-1.1* and *kal-1.2*, and these have been used to study the effects on GnRH development, using GnRH-1 and GnRH-3 green fluorescent protein (GFP) fusions to model the migratory behaviour of GnRH-1- and GnRH-3-expressing neurons. Antisense knockdown of *kal-1.1* inhibited migration of both hypothalamic and terminal nerve GnRH neurons into the pre-optic area, causing these to accumulate in the olfactory region and dorsal telencephalon [22]. GnRH-3 neuronal migration from the olfactory regions to the forebrain was also supressed and an overall change in body cavity size could be seen. Knockdown of *kal-1.1* had no apparent phenotypes in the migration of these populations of cells, indicating slight differences from the zebrafish model system [22].

Drosophila kal-1

D. melanogaster is used along with several other genetically tractable organisms to identify and characterise pathways and genes that share common functions across species to model key biological processes in humans. Although *Drosophila* has a number of similar genes to the GnRH receptor, it has no GnRH system. *Drosophila* does, however, have one *kal-1* ortholog, encoding a protein that is smaller than vertebrate and worm anosmins [20]. The *D. melanogaster* Kal gene *(DmKal-1)* has a WAP domain and two FnIII repeats [20]; the C-terminal region has low similarity with the third (32%) and the fourth (36%) human FnIII repeats [36]. *DmKal-1* is expressed in the second half of embryogenesis during morphogenetic processes of germ band retraction, dorsal closure and head involution (HI), and shows a dynamic and complex expression pattern [37].

Interestingly, gonadal *kal-1* expression was limited to the posterior part of the male gonad in the position where the male-specific somatic gonadal precursors are located; the first time that expression of a *kal-1* ortholog was demonstrated to be sex specific, and making the transcript a useful tool for studying sex determination in the gonad. Expression of *kal-1* within the cells of the antennal organ implies a chemosensory function and suggests that the role of anosmin-1 during olfactory development is conserved between vertebrates and invertebrates [37].

DmKal-1 is also strongly expressed in the ectodermal cells of the mandibular segment, and these function in the formation of the head skeleton of the *Drosophila* embryo. Using UAS/Gal4 to drive overexpression, and to potentially model the head/craniofacial abnormalities seen in KS, *DmKal-1* was produced in a number of different tissues. Modified *DmKal-1* protein isoforms, representing mutations found in KS patients, were overexpressed in developing head regions and qualitative differences in the phenotypes induced by the expression of the different mutant forms were measured [36]. Several of the *DmKal-1* mutants caused strong alterations in the

Table 4. *Drosophila* protein overexpression, GAL4 drivers and phenotypes

Mutant	Description	Phenotype
UAS-Dm*Kal-1[W200-STOP]*; *179y*-GAL4	C-terminal truncated protein FnIII-1 and other FnIII domains	no effect on morphogenesis
UAS-Dm*Kal-1[Q421-STOP]*; *179y*-GAL4	missing a putative heparan sulphate binding site	no effect on morphogenesis
UAS-*kal-1 [H384-STOP]*; *179y*-GAL4	C-terminal deletion	no effect on morphogenesis
UAS-*kal-1[N236K]*; *179y*-GAL4	mutation mimics those affecting GnRH-1 neuronal migration	mouth hook defects, lack of sclerotization and HI defects
UAS-*kal-1 [C127/128S+N236K]*	mutation in WAP domain suppresses N236K	no phenotype

Adapted from Andrenacci et al. [37].

cephalopharyngeal skeleton of the larva, when these were overexpressed in cells surrounding the head skeleton, supporting a role for *DmKal-1* in head morphogenesis (table 4).

Several C-terminally truncated proteins, missing part of the first FnIII domain and all the other FnIII domains, or missing heparan sulphate binding sites had no effect on head morphogenesis when overexpressed – indicating that the C-terminal domain of *DmKal-1* is not needed for head morphogenesis, although protein instability caused by truncation could not be ruled out as a cause for lack of phenotype. In addition, a mutation *(kal-1-N236K)* in the FnIII-1 domain, which mimics a human KAL-1 mutation affecting GnRH-1 cell migration [17], produced major head alterations, abnormal median tooth development, mouth hook defects, a skeleton with a less sclerotized structure, and HI defects. Further, to determine whether the WAP domain was essential for alterations in the HI process induced by the N236K substitution, a double substitution C-S was introduced in the four-disulphide core motif both in the wild-type protein and N236K mutant. This UAS-*kal-1[C127/128S+N236K]* mutant suppressed the HI phenotype induced by the N236K substitution [36].

Nematode *kal-1*

The *C. elegans Kal-1* ortholog *(Kal-1)* has proven especially useful in studying the relative roles of the WAP and FnIII domains found in 'anosmins'. *Kal-1* has six exons, encoding a secreted protein of 700 amino acids that shares 36% overall similarity with its human ortholog. In common with human *KAL1*, it contains a cysteine-rich region, a WAP-like protease inhibitor domain followed by four FnIII domains, indicating that an ancestral gene with a sequence and domain organization similar to KAL-1 was present before the separation of invertebrates and vertebrates [38].

Expression Pattern and of kal-1 during Embryogenesis

The sites of expression of *kal-1* were characterized by means of a transcriptional reporter, encoding GFP fused to 5.3 kb of 5′ upstream *kal-1* promoter sequence. Expression of the *kal-1-gfp* transcription reporter was first detected in embryos at around the 50-cell stage in 2–3 cells, widening during the 'comma' stage of embryonic development to neuroblast cells in the developing head and tail ganglia, and motor neurons in the ventral nerve cord and mid-body regions. Expression was also observed in the excretory and uterine cells during the larval stages and throughout adulthood [20]. A group of 8–10 neuroblasts are descendants of the AB blastomere, located on the ventral surface of the embryo, and these cells initially surround and later close the gap left by gastrulation. KAL-1 secreted by these cells may act as a substrate for epithelial migration when these cells migrate round the embryo to join at the ventral midline for ventral enclosure [38].

Loss of Function of kal-1

Two independently obtained deletion alleles of *kal-1* predicted to represent molecular null alleles display defects in ventral neuroblast migration during embryonic development, resulting in a delay of closure of the gastrulation cleft [40]. These defects are mild and resemble loss of function mutants of ephrin signalling in *C. elegans* [40]. The double mutants between ephrin mutants and *kal-1* result in strongly enhanced phenotypes, suggesting that *kal-1* and ephrin signalling serve redundant functions during ventral neuroblast migration [40].

Larval stages and adult worms of *kal-1* null mutants show incompletely penetrant defects in epidermal morphogenesis [38, 40]. The cellular basis of this abnormality was analysed by visualizing epithelial cell boundaries during the ventral enclosure process using rhodaminated phalloidin staining and by staining adherens junctions at later stages using JAM-1 monoclonal antibodies. For both loss-of-function and overexpressing *kal-1* mutants, epidermal cells differentiate correctly but migrate and form abnormal reciprocal contacts in the mutant embryos. Cells that normally join at the midline and form a stereotypical symmetrical pattern in wild-type embryos instead form clustered irregular shapes and abnormal/ectopic contacts in mutant embryos [38].

Kal-1 mutants did not show significant differences from wild types with respect to sensory behaviours [38]. Consistent with this observation, as far as they have been analysed, the *kal-1* mutants display only mild neuro-anatomical defects, e.g. an extra branching defect in male-specific EF3 dendrites [38]. Together with the results in regard to epidermal morphogenesis, this raises the possibility that *kal-1* may also act redundantly with as of yet unknown genetic pathways in neural development.

Table 5. *kal-1* mutant genotypes and phenotypes with rescue

Genotype	Percent normal male tail phenotype	Notes
kal-1(gb503);him-8 (e1489)	18.1	loss of function
kal-1(gb503); him-8 (e1489); gbEx10	68.2	rescue with kal-1 (genomic)
kal-1(gb503); him-8 (e1489); gbEx13b	59.0	rescue with *C. elegans kal-1* (cDNA)
kal-1(gb503); him-8 (e1489); gbEx17a	48.9	rescue with human *KAL1* (cDNA)

Adapted from Rugarli et al. [38].

Human KAL1 Gene Is Functionally Conserved in C. elegans

In *C. elegans*, the most penetrant of the phenotypes observed in *kal-1* mutants were tail ray abnormalities (table 5). These tail abnormalities ranged from altered shape to extra or reduced sensory ray numbers, but in this specific instance did not cause any change in the ability of males to reproduce. Male tail defects were largely rescued in mutant *gb503* worms carrying a cosmid with the complete genomic sequence of *kal-1*, both by the *kal-1* cDNA control and by the human *KAL-1* cDNA – also driven by *kal-1* regulatory sequences. Overexpression of the human sequence caused defects very similar to those caused by the *C. elegans* sequence. These results confirm the functional affinity between human and *C. elegans kal-1*, in addition to the genomic and protein similarities [38, 39].

Molecular Basis for kal-1 Function

Several proteins and extracellular matrix molecules interact with *kal-1* to mediate its function in vivo [18–20, 40]. Overexpression of *kal-1* in vivo has been useful in modelling the effects of mutations in KAL-1 on cellular morphogenesis and in dissecting the functions of the individual domains encoded by *kal-1* [20].

Before the studies in *C. elegans*, not much was known about factors interacting with *kal-1* in vivo, the individual domain functions, or the gene pathways upstream and downstream of *kal-1*. The *C. elegans* anosmin has distinct functions with respect to neuronal branching and routing, shown by overexpression of *kal-1* in vivo [20]. In AIY interneurons, *kal-1* is downstream of the *ttx-3* transcription factor, and transgenic nematodes overexpressing *kal-1* under control of an AIY-specific *ttx-3* promoter fragment have prominent axon branching defects (table 6). This phenotype could not be reproduced by overexpression of other extracellular cell adhesion molecules under the same conditions, or by overexpression of mutations within the C-terminal and FnIII domains of *kal-1*, including one analogous to the human N267K missense mutation seen in patients with X-KS. In contrast, the axonal branching phenotype was still seen when overexpressing a variant with a mutation in the WAP domain – suggestive of a separate function for the WAP domain and the first fibronectin domain

Table 6. *kal-1* mutant neuronal phenotypes

Overexpression genotype	Neuronal phenotype	Comments
Vector	AIY branching (3%)	control
ttx-3::kal-1	AIY branching (87%)	branching defect
ttx-3::kal-1ΔC-terminal	AIY branching (8%)	no branching defect (*ΔC-terminal* mimics truncating KS mutation)
ttx-3::kal-1S241K (FnIII-1)	AIY branching (7%)	no branching defect (*S241K* mimics N267K KS mutation)
ttx-3::kal-1mWAP	AIY branching: extensive arborisation (85%)	qualitatively different branching defect (*mWAP* mimics KS mutations in WAP domain)
unc-119::kal-1	AFD misrouting (51%)	wild-type protein
unc-119::kal-1S241K	AFD misrouting (45%)	no significant difference in branching defect from wild type
unc-119::kal-1mWAP	AFD misrouting (26%)	difference in branching defect from wild type

Adapted from Bülow et al. [20].

in vivo. Pan-neuronal overexpression of *kal-1* under control of a pan-neuronal *unc-119* promoter, led to a separate axonal routing defect, which was unchanged by the FnIII mutant (S241K). However, lower numbers of axon branching defective neurons were observed in overexpressors of the WAP mutant (mWAP) [20] (table 6).

As the KAL-1 S241K mutant protein (analogous to the N267K anosmin-1 mutation) appeared to be neither mislocalized nor unstable, these data indicated that the axonal branching phenotype in AIY interneurons was highly specific for KAL-1/anosmin-1. Thus, the axon branching phenotype presented a bioassay to interrogate *kal-1* function in vivo. Using this bioassay in a forward genetic screen, the authors isolated a number of suppressor mutants that were required for the expression of the *kal-1*-dependent axon branching phenotype [20]. Conceptually, such suppressor mutants could either be generic suppressors of axonal branches or, they could be specific for the *kal-1*-dependent branches. The authors found, that the isolated mutants could only suppress the axon branching phenotype elicited by *kal-1* expression in AIY interneurons, but could not suppress branches in AIY interneurons elicited by other genetic manipulations [20]. Consequently, the suppressor mutations are specific for the *kal-1*-dependent branching phenotype and, by inference, the affected genes may be important for *kal-1*-dependent signalling.

Studies of Heparan Sulphate Interactions with Nematode Anosmin Reveal Potential IHH Candidate Genes

Molecular cloning of the suppressor mutants identified through the axon branching bioassay, led to the discovery of mutations in *hst-6*, the sole *C. elegans* gene coding for a heparan sulphate 6-O-sulphotransferase [20, 41], in *hse-5*, the *C. elegans* gene coding for the heparan sulphate C5 glucuronic acid epimerase [20, 41], and in *pst-1*, which codes for an intracellular phosphoadenosyl-phosphosulphate transporter [42]. All three gene proteins are involved in the modification of heparan sulphate, an extracellular polysaccharide (see below). Strikingly, loss of *hst-6*, *hse-5* and, *pst-1* function in vivo also caused midline crossover defects of ventral cord neurons [41], reminiscent of the corticospinal tract decussation defects thought to underpin mirror movements in X-KS [12–15].

The above data demonstrate that, in vivo, *kal-1* requires heparan sulphate sugars with specific modifications to exert its function. These findings are in accord with biochemical studies. First, KAL-1 protein appears to physically interact with heparan sulphate proteoglycans in *C. elegans* [40]. Second, the binding of anosmin-1 to cells in culture could be competed by the addition of heparin (a highly sulphated form of heparan sulphate) or by high salt concentration [20, 43]. Finally, physical binding of anosmin-1 to the fibroblast growth factor receptor (FGFR1) could be modulated by the exogenous addition of heparin [44].

Heparan sulphates are unbranched polysaccharides of the extracellular space which are attached to a protein core that can either be secreted or membrane-bound [45]. Their sugar chains are characterized by alternating hexuronic acid and N-acetyl-glucosamine residues. During synthesis in the Golgi apparatus, the sugar chains undergo a number of non-random and non-uniform modifications that define a domain structure within the sugar chain [46]. These domains are comprised of complex sugar modification patterns including sulphations and epimerizations of the sugar residues and provide binding sites for interacting proteins [47]. By way of their modification patterns, the heparan sulphate sugars are believed to be involved in mediating and regulating cell-cell communication, particularly during development of the nervous system, by modulating how ligands interact with their receptors [48–52].

One of the best understood examples of heparan sulphate function is its role in FGF signalling. It was demonstrated that different heparan sulphate oligosaccharides of similar length could elicit differential responses in a cell culture assay for FGF function, indicating that specific modifications within the heparan sulphate sugar chain may be crucial for defining FGF signalling [53]. And second, crystal structures of the FGF receptor and its FGF ligand in conjunction with heparin showed that specific sulphate residues on the heparin sugar chain interact with defined amino acid residues of the FGF receptor as well as the FGF ligand [reviewed in 54]. Not surprisingly, mutations in the genes encoding both FGFR1 and its ligand

FGF8 have also been shown to underlie KS and nIHH [55–57]. Furthermore, work in *C. elegans* genes hints at the significance of heparan sulphate modifications in *kal-1* function [20]. Thus, both in vivo and in vitro evidence now implicate heparan sulphate sugar chains and their modification patterns with two known genetic pathways that, when mutated, can cause IHH namely *KAL1* and *FGFR1/FGF8*. It will thus be an important avenue of future research to investigate whether the human orthologs of the heparan sulphate-related genes identified in the nematode *C. elegans* may underlie those cases of KS and nIHH whose basis remains to date genetically elusive [58].

Conclusions

Orthologs and paralogs of *kal-1* are found in widely different genera and species, including a few genetically tractable species of fish, fruit flies and nematodes (fig. 1). These appear to share common interacting genetic and biochemical pathways, and their genetic manipulation has demonstrated a number of striking similarities with the phenotypes observed in humans, including, cranial anomalies, GnRH-1 neuronal migration defects and axonal routing abnormalities. Although these morphological changes are artificially induced in the laboratory, the various studies all indicate a strong conservation of *kal-1* function over species, thus allowing a more detailed analysis of *kal-1* domain function and of similar mutations in vivo that would be possible in vitro. In particular, the work showing rescue of *C. elegans kal-1* mutants with human *KAL1* further supports conservation of function between species. Thus, in answer to the question of what other genes could underlie KS and or nIHH, important leads may come from work that originated in *C. elegans*.

References

1 Quinton R, Duke VM, de Zoysa PA, Platts AD, Valentine A, Kendall B, Pickman S, Kirk JM, Besser GM, Jacobs HS, Bouloux PM: The neuroradiology of Kallmann's syndrome: a genotypic and phenotypic analysis. J Clin Endocrinol Metab 1996;81:3010–3017.

2 Quinton R, Duke VM, Robertson A, Kirk JM, Matfin G, de Zoysa PA, Azcona C, MacColl GS, Jacobs HS, Conway GS, Besser GM, Stanhope RG, Bouloux PM: Idiopathic gonadotrophin deficiency: genetic questions addressed through phenotypic characterization. Clin Endocrinol (Oxf) 2001;55:163–174.

3 Pitteloud N, Hayes FJ, Boepple PA, DeCruz S, Seminara SB, MacLaughlin DT, Crowley WF Jr: The role of prior pubertal development, biochemical markers of testicular maturation, and genetics in elucidating the phenotypic heterogeneity of idiopathic hypogonadotropic hypogonadism. J Clin Endocrinol Metab 2002;87:152–160.

4 Franco B, Guioli S, Pragliola A, Incerti B, Bardoni B, Tonlorenzi R, Carrozzo R, Maestrini E, Pieretti M, Taillon-Miller P, Brown CJ, Willard HF, Lawrence C, Persico MG, Camerino G, Ballabio A: A gene deleted in Kallmann's syndrome shares homology with neural cell adhesion and axonal path-finding molecules. Nature 1991;353:529–536.

5 Legouis R, Hardelin JP, Levilliers J, Claverie JM, Compain S, Wunderle V, Millasseau P, Le Paslier D, Cohen D, Caterina D, Bougueleret L, Delemarre-Van de Waal, Lutfalla G, Wessenbach J, Petit C: The candidate gene for the X-linked Kallmann syndrome encodes a protein related to adhesion molecules. Cell 1991;67:423–435.
6 Schwanzel-Fukuda M, Bick D, Pfaff DW: Luteinizing hormone-releasing hormone (LHRH)-expressing cells do not migrate normally in an inherited hypogonadal (Kallmann) syndrome. Brain Res Mol Brain Res 1989;6:311–626.
7 Salenave S, Chanson P, Bry H, Pugeat M, Cabrol S, Carel JC, Murat A, Lecomte P, Brailly S, Hardelin JP, Dode C, Young J: Kallmann's syndrome: a comparison of the reproductive phenotypes in men carrying KAL1 and FGFR1/KAL2 mutations. J Clin Endocrinol Metab 2008;93:758–763.
8 Parenti G, Rizzolo MG, Ghezzi M, Di Maio S, Sperandeo MP, Incerti B, Franco B, Ballabio A, Andria G: Variable penetrance of hypogonadism in a sibship with Kallmann syndrome due to a deletion of the KAL gene. Am J Med Genet 1995;57:476–478.
9 Ribeiro RS, Vieira TC, Abucham J: Reversible Kallmann syndrome: report of the first case with a KAL1 mutation and literature review. Eur J Endocrinol 2007;156; 285–290.
10 Soussi-Yanicostas N, de Castro F, Julliard AK, Perfettini I, Chédotal A, Petit C: Anosmin-1, defective in the X-linked form of Kallmann syndrome, promotes axonal branch formation from olfactory bulb output neurons. Cell 2002;109:217–228.
11 MacColl GS, Quinton R, Bouloux PM: GnRH neuronal development: insights into hypogonadotrophic hypogonadism. Trends Endocrinol Metab 2002;13:112–118.
12 Mayston MJ, Harrison LM, Quinton R, Stephens JA, Krams M, Bouloux PM: Mirror movements in X-linked Kallmann's syndrome. I. A neurophysiological study. Brain 1997;120:1199–1216.
13 Krams M, Quinton R, Mayston MJ, Harrison LM, Dolan RJ, Bouloux PM, Stephens JA, Frackowiak RS, Passingham RE: Mirror movements in X-linked Kallmann's syndrome. II. A PET study. Brain 1997; 120:1217–1228.
14 Krams M, Quinton R, Ashburner J, Friston KJ, Frackowiak RS, Bouloux PM, Passingham RE: Kallmann's syndrome: mirror movements associated with bilateral corticospinal tract hypertrophy. Neurology 1999;52:816–822.
15 Farmer SF, Harrison LM, Mayston MJ, Parekh A, James LM, Stephens JA: Abnormal cortex-muscle interactions in subjects with X-linked Kallmann's syndrome and mirror movements. Brain 2004;127: 385–397.
16 Robertson A, MacColl GS, Nash JA, Boehm MK, Perkins SJ, Bouloux PM: Molecular modelling and experimental studies of mutation and cell-adhesion sites in the fibronectin type III and whey acidic protein domains of human anosmin-1. Biochem J 2001; 357:647–659.
17 Cariboni A, Pimpinelli F, Colamarino S, Zaninetti R, Piccolella M, Rumio C, Piva F, Rugarli EI, Maggi R: The product of X-linked Kallmann's syndrome gene (KAL1) affects the migratory activity of gonadotropin-releasing hormone (GnRH)-producing neurons. Hum Mol Genet 2004;13:2781–2791.
18 Hu Y, González-Martínez D, Kim SH, Bouloux PM: Cross-talk of anosmin-1, the protein implicated in X-linked Kallmann's syndrome, with heparan sulphate and urokinase-type plasminogen activator. Biochem J 2004;384:495–505.
19 González-Martínez D, Kim SH, Hu Y, Guimond S, Schofield J, Winyard P, Vannelli GB, Turnbull J, Bouloux PM: Anosmin-1 modulates fibroblast growth factor receptor 1 signaling in human gonadotropin-releasing hormone olfactory neuroblasts through a heparan sulfate-dependent mechanism. J Neurosci 2004;24:10384–10392.
20 Bülow HE, Berry KL, Topper LH, Peles E, Hobert O: Heparan sulfate proteoglycan-dependent induction of axon branching and axon misrouting by the Kallmann syndrome gene kal-1. Proc Natl Acad Sci USA 2002;99:6346–6351.
21 Whitlock KE, Smith KM, Kim H, Harden MV: A role for foxd3 and sox10 in the differentiation of gonadotropin-releasing hormone (GnRH) cells in the zebrafish Danio rerio. Development 2005;132: 5491–5502.
22 Okubo K, Sakai F, Lau EL, Yoshizaki G, Takeuchi Y, Naruse K, Aida K, Nagahama Y: Forebrain gonadotropin-releasing hormone neuronal development: insights from transgenic medaka and the relevance to X-linked Kallmann syndrome. Endocrinology 2006;147:1076–1084.
23 Schwanzel-Fukuda M, Pfaff DW: Origin of luteinizing hormone-releasing hormone neurons. Nature 1989;338:161–164.
24 Wray S, Grant P, Gainer H: Evidence that cells expressing luteinizing hormone-releasing hormone mRNA in the mouse are derived from progenitor cells in the olfactory placode. Proc Natl Acad Sci USA 1989;86:8132–8136.
25 Keverne EB: Pheromones, vomeronasal function, and gender-specific behavior. Cell 2002;108:735–738.
26 Wray S: Molecular mechanisms for migration of placodally derived GnRH neurons. Chem Senses 2002;27:569–572.

27 Tobet SA, Schwarting GA: Minireview: recent progress in gonadotropin-releasing hormone neuronal migration. Endocrinology 2006;147:1159–1165.
28 Duke VM, Winyard PJ, Thorogood P, Soothill P, Bouloux PM, Woolf AS: KAL, a gene mutated in Kallmann's syndrome, is expressed in the first trimester of human development. Mol Cell Endocrinol 1995;110:73–79.
29 Hardelin JP, Julliard AK, Moniot B, Soussi-Yanicostas N, Verney C, Schwanzel-Fukuda M, Ayer-Le Lievre C, Petit C: Anosmin-1 is a regionally restricted component of basement membranes and interstitial matrices during organogenesis: implications for the developmental anomalies of X chromosome-linked Kallmann syndrome. Dev Dyn 1999;215:26–44.
30 MacColl GS, Bouloux PM, Quinton R: Kallmann syndrome: adhesion, afferents, and anosmia. Neuron 2002;34:675–678.
31 Ardouin O, Legouis R, Fasano L, David-Watine B, Korn H, Hardelin J, Petit C: Characterization of the two zebrafish orthologues of the KAL-1 gene underlying X chromosome-linked Kallmann syndrome. Mech Dev 2000;90:89–94.
32 Legouis R, Lievre CA, Leibovici M, Lapointe F, Petit C: Expression of the KAL gene in multiple neuronal sites during chicken development. Proc Natl Acad Sci USA 1993;90:2461–2465.
33 Lutz B, Kuratani S, Rugarli EI, Wawersik S, Wong C, Bieber FR, Ballabio A, Eichele G: Expression of the Kallmann syndrome gene in human fetal brain and in the manipulated chick embryo. Hum Mol Genet 1994;3:1717–1723.
34 Ernest S, Guadagnini S, Prevost MC, Soussi-Yanicostas N: Localization of anosmin-1a and anosmin-1b in the inner ear and neuromasts of zebrafish. Gene Expr Patterns 2007;7:274–281.
35 Yanicostas C, Ernest S, Dayraud C, Petit C, Soussi-Yanicostas N: Essential requirement for zebrafish anosmin-1a in the migration of the posterior lateral line primordium. Dev Biol 2008;320:469–479.
36 Andrenacci D, Grimaldi MR, Panetta V, Riano E, Rugarli EI, Graziani F: Functional dissection of the Drosophila Kallmann's syndrome protein DmKal-1. BMC Genet 2006;7:47–61.
37 Andrenacci D, Le Bras S, Rosaria Grimaldi M, Rugarli E, Graziani F: Embryonic expression pattern of the Drosophila Kallmann syndrome gene kal-1. Gene Expr Patterns 2004;5:67–73.
38 Rugarli EI, Di Schiavi E, Hilliard MA, Arbucci S, Ghezzi C, Facciolli A, Coppola G, Ballabio A, Bazzicalupo P: The Kallmann syndrome gene homolog in *C. elegans* is involved in epidermal morphogenesis and neurite branching. Development 2002;129:1283–1294.
39 Lints R, Emmons SW: Regulation of sex-specific differentiation and mating behavior in *C. elegans* by a new member of the DM domain transcription factor family. Genes Dev 2002;16:2390–2402.
40 Hudson ML, Kinnunen T, Cinar HN, Chisholm AD: *C. elegans* Kallmann syndrome protein KAL-1 interacts with syndecan and glypican to regulate neuronal cell migrations. Dev Biol 2006;294:352–365.
41 Bülow HE, Hobert O: Differential sulfations and epimerization define heparan sulfate specificity in nervous system development. Neuron 2004;41:723–736.
42 Bhattacharya R, Townley RA, Berry KL, Bülow HE: The PAPS transporter PST-1 is required for heparan sulfation and is essential for viability and neural development in C. elegans. J Cell Sci 2009;122:4492–4504.
43 Soussi-Yanicostas N, Faivre-Sarrailh C, Hardelin JP, Levilliers J, Rougon, G, Petit C: Anosmin-1 underlying the X chromosome-linked Kallmann syndrome is an adhesion molecule that can modulate neurite growth in a cell-type specific manner. J Cell Sci 1998;111:2953–2965.
44 Hu Y, Guimond SE, Travers P, Cadman SM, Hohenester E, Turnbull JE, Kim SH, Bouloux PM: Novel mechanism of fibroblast growth factor receptor 1 regulation by extracellular matrix protein anosmin-1. J Biol Chem 2009;284 :29905–29920.
45 Bernfield M, Gotte M, Park PW, Reizes O, Fitzgerald ML, Lincecum J, Zako M: Functions of cell surface heparan sulfate proteoglycans. Annu Rev Biochem 1999;68:729–777.
46 Lindahl U, Kusche-Gullberg M, Kjellen L: Regulated diversity of heparan sulfate. J Biol Chem 1998;273: 24979–24982.
47 Esko JD, Selleck SB: Order out of chaos: assembly of ligand binding sites in heparan sulfate. Annu Rev Biochem 2002;71:435–471.
48 Bülow HE, Hobert O: The molecular diversity of glycosaminoglycans shapes animal development. Ann Rev Cell Dev Biol 2006;22:375–407.
49 Bülow HE, Tjoe N, Townley RA, Didiano D, van Kuppevelt TH, Hobert O: Extracellular sugar modifications provide instructive and cell-specific information for axon-guidance choices. Curr Biol 2008; 18:1978–1985.
50 Holt CE, Dickson BJ: Sugar codes for axons? Neuron 2005;46:169–172.
51 Lee JS, Chien CB: When sugars guide axons: insights from heparan sulphate proteoglycan mutants. Nat Rev Genet 2004;5:923–935.
52 Van Vactor D, Wall DP, Johnson KG: Heparan sulfate proteoglycans and the emergence of neuronal connectivity. Curr Opin Neurobiol 2006;16:40–51.

53 Guimond SE, Turnbull JE: Fibroblast growth factor receptor signalling is dictated by specific heparan sulphate saccharides. Curr Biol 2006;9:1343–1346.
54 Pellegrini L: Role of heparan sulfate in fibroblast growth factor signalling: a structural view. Curr Opin Struct Biol 2001;11:629–634.
55 Dodé C, Levilliers J, Dupont JM, De Paepe A, Le Dû N, Soussi-Yanicostas N, Coimbra RS, Delmaghani S, Compain-Nouaille S, Baverel F, Pêcheux C, Le Tessier D, Cruaud C, Delpech M, Speleman F, Vermeulen S, Amalfitano A, Bachelot Y, Bouchard P, Cabrol S, Carel JC, Delemarre-van de Waal H, Goulet-Salmon B, Kottler ML, Richard O, Sanchez-Franco F, Saura R, Young J, Petit C, Hardelin JP: Loss-of-function mutations in FGFR1 cause autosomal dominant Kallmann syndrome. Nat Genet 2003;33:463–465.
56 Pitteloud N, Acierno JS Jr, Meysing A, Eliseenkova AV, Ma J, Ibrahimi OA, Metzger DL, Hayes FJ, Dwyer AA, Hughes VA, Yialamas M, Hall JE, Grant E, Mohammadi M, Crowley WF Jr. Mutations in fibroblast growth factor receptor 1 cause both Kallmann syndrome and normosmic idiopathic hypogonadotropic hypogonadism. Proc Natl Acad Sci USA 2006;103:6281–6286.
57 Falardeau J, Chung WC, Beenken A, Raivio T, Plummer L, Sidis Y, Jacobson-Dickman EE, Eliseenkova AV, Ma J, Dwyer A, Quinton R, Na S, Hall JE, Huot C, Alois N, Pearce SH, Cole LW, Hughes V, Mohammadi M, Tsai P, Pitteloud N: Decreased FGF8 signaling causes deficiency of gonadotropin-releasing hormone in humans and mice. J Clin Invest 2008;118:2822–2831.
58 Crowley WF, Pitteloud N, Seminara S: New genes controlling human reproduction and how you find them. Trans Am Clin Climatol Assoc 2008;119:29–38.
59 Maya-Nuñez G, Zenteno JC, Ulloa-Aguirre A, Kofman-Alfaro S, Mendez JP: A recurrent missense mutation in the KAL gene in patients with X-linked Kallmann's syndrome. J Clin Endocrinol Metab 1998;83:1650–1653.
60 Georgopoulos NA, Koika V, Galli-Tsinopoulou A, Spiliotis BE, Adonakis G, Keramida MK, Sgourou A, Koufogiannis KD, Papachatzopoulou A, Papavassiliou AG, Kourounis G, Vagenakis GA: Renal dysgenesis and KAL1 gene defects in patients with sporadic Kallmann syndrome. Fertil Steril 2007;88:1311–1317.
61 Oliveira LM, Seminara SB, Beranova M, Hayes FJ, Valkenburgh SB, Schipani E, Costa EM, Latronico AC, Crowley WF Jr, Vallejo M: The importance of autosomal genes in Kallmann syndrome: genotype-phenotype correlations and neuroendocrine characteristics. J Clin Endocrinol Metab 2001;86:1532–1538.
62 Albuisson J, Pêcheux C, Carel JC, Lacombe D, Leheup B, Lapuzina P, Bouchard P, Legius E, Matthijs G, Wasniewska M, Delpech M, Young J, Hardelin JP, Dodé C: Kallmann syndrome: 14 novel mutations in KAL1 and FGFR1 (KAL2). Hum Mutat 2005;25:98–99.
63 Gamble JA, Karunadasa DK, Pape JR, Skynner MJ, Todman MG, Bicknell RJ, Allen JP, Herbison AE: Disruption of ephrin signaling associates with disordered axophilic migration of the gonadotropin-releasing hormone neurons. J Neurosci 2005;25:3142–3150.
64 Schwarting GA, Kostek C, Bless EP, Ahmad N, Tobet SA: Deleted in colorectal cancer (DCC) regulates the migration of luteinizing hormone-releasing hormone neurons to the basal forebrain. J Neurosci 2001;21:911–919.
65 Schwarting GA, Raitcheva D, Bless EP, Ackerman SL, Tobet S: Netrin 1-mediated chemoattraction regulates the migratory pathway of LHRH neurons. Eur J Neurosci 2004;19:11–20.
66 Chung WC, Moyle SS, Tsai PS: Fibroblast growth factor 8 signaling through fibroblast growth factor receptor 1 is required for the emergence of gonadotropin-releasing hormone neurons. Endocrinology 2008;149:4997–5003.

Richard Quinton, MA, MD, FRCP
Consultant and Senior Lecturer in Endocrinology
Endocrine Research Group, Institute of Human Genetics, University of Newcastle-upon-Tyne
Newcastle-upon-Tyne NE1 3BZ (UK)
Tel. +44 191 2824635, Fax +44 191 2820129, E-Mail richard.quinton@ncl.ac.uk

Quinton R (ed): Kallmann Syndrome and Hypogonadotropic Hypogonadism.
Front Horm Res. Basel, Karger, 2010, vol 39, pp 78–93

Biological Actions and Interactions of Anosmin-1

Catherine Choy · Soo-Hyun Kim

Division of Basic Medical Sciences, St. George's Medical School, University of London, London, UK

Abstract

Kallmann syndrome is a multigenic human developmental disorder where the molecular pathogenesis is still only partially understood and there is no single unifying animal model. The protein anosmin-1, encoded by the *KAL1* gene, is associated with the X-linked form of the disease. The biology and molecular structure of anosmin-1 has been investigated systematically over the years by various cell culture experiments, biochemical analyses and animal models. Anosmin-1 is an extracellular matrix-associated protein which plays pleiotropic roles in neuronal development, migration and organogenesis.

When idiopathic hypogonadotropic hypogonadism (IHH) is combined with anosmia or hypoanosmia, it is defined as Kallmann syndrome (KS). KS is a relatively rare congenital heterogeneous disorder, affecting approximately 1 in 8,000 males [1] and with a 3- to 5-fold excess of male cases over female reported by most investigators. The association of hypothalamic gonadotropin-releasing hormone (GnRH) deficiency and olfactory bulb (OB) dysgenesis is presumably caused by the disruption of the olfactory GnRH neuronal migration during early embryogenesis [2]. KS can be transmitted monogenically in either X-linked, autosomal dominant or autosomal recessive modes of inheritance, but the majority of cases are sporadic. However, recent studies have highlighted the more complex nature of the genetics of this disease [3, 4]. So far, six different factors have been identified as the underlying genetic defects: anosmin-1 *(KAL1)* [5, 6], fibroblast growth factor receptor 1 *(FGFR1)* [7] and its ligand *(FGF8)* [10], prokineticin 2 *(PROK2)* and its receptor *(PROKR2)* [8], and chromodomain helicase DNA binding protein 7 *(CHD7)* [9]. However, the genetic basis of the majority of cases probably still remains unaccounted for. KS is thus an oligogenic trait involving a number of key signaling pathways, with further genetic defects remaining to be discovered.

KAL1 was first identified as the genetic locus for X-linked KS nearly two decades ago [5, 6]. During this period, the exact function and regulation of the *KAL1* gene and its encoded protein named anosmin-1 have been the focus of much research. The *KAL1* gene localised to Xp22.3, contains 14 exons encompassing 220 kb of genomic DNA and 2,043 bases of coding sequences. *KAL1* orthologs have been identified or predicted in many vertebrates and invertebrates including fruit fly, worm, chicken, dog, fish, frog, monkey and chimpanzee [11]. Despite full sequencing of the mouse genome, an ortholog remains unidentified, potentially due to such significant sequence divergence from human that the value of any mouse model would anyway be severely limited. However, studies using *Caenorhabditis elegans*, zebrafish, medaka and *Drosophila melanogaster* have provided substantial new information. Furthermore, the sequence alignment of known *KAL1* genes shows high levels of homology involving specific protein domains, suggesting important functions of these regions (fig. 1). This review will focus on several recent studies providing significant new insights into the functions of anosmin-1, in particular its molecular structure, biological activities and interacting partners that may assist or enable its function. Other KS-associated molecules and the complex nature of the phenotype-genotype relations in KS will be reviewed in separate chapters of this volume.

Molecular Structure of the Functional Domains of Anosmin-1

The open reading frame of human *KAL1* cDNA encodes a 680-amino acid protein with a conceptual molecular weight of 74 kDa, which subsequently undergoes N-glycosylation contributing to an observed molecular weight of 85–100 kDa of the mature protein [12–14]. There has been no direct confirmation regarding which of the putative glycosylation sites are involved in this post-translational modification. However, it has been shown that glycosylation has an eminent role in functional protein folding and secretion, as well as other protein binding interactions in cellular signalling events [15]. Intracellular localisation studies have demonstrated that anosmin-1 is an extracellular matrix (ECM)-associated secretory protein, showing accumulation along the plasma membrane and within endoplasmic vesicles, as well as in the surrounding medium scattering to adjacent cells [16, 17]. These observations are consistent with the lack of any hydrophobic transmembrane domains or glycosyl phosphotidyl inositol anchorage site in the structure of anosmin-1. Instead, it comprises a signal peptide, a cysteine-rich N-terminal region, a whey acid protein (WAP)-like four-disulphide core motif, followed by four tandem fibronectin type III (FnIII)-like domains and a histidine-rich C-terminus (fig. 1).

The WAP domain in anosmin-1 contains four-disulphide core motif, similar to those found in secretory leukocyte protease inhibitor, elafin, human secretory protein 4 (HE4), Westmead DMBA8 nonmetastatic cDNA 1 (WDNM1) and 20-kDa prostate stromal protein (ps20). Secretory leukocyte protease inhibitor and elafin are anti-serine protease and anti-microbial molecules with a role in innate immune defence, wound healing and tissue remodelling, and elafin degrades ECM proteins such as

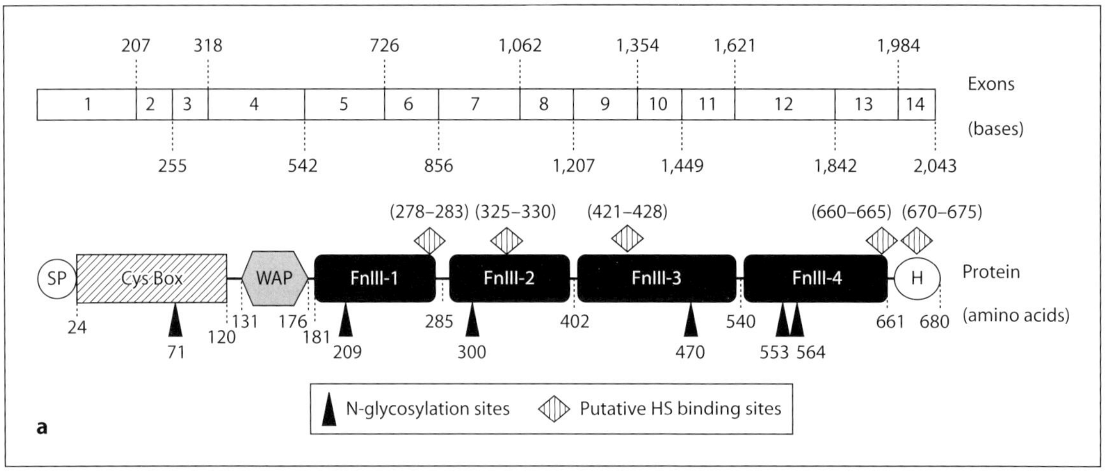

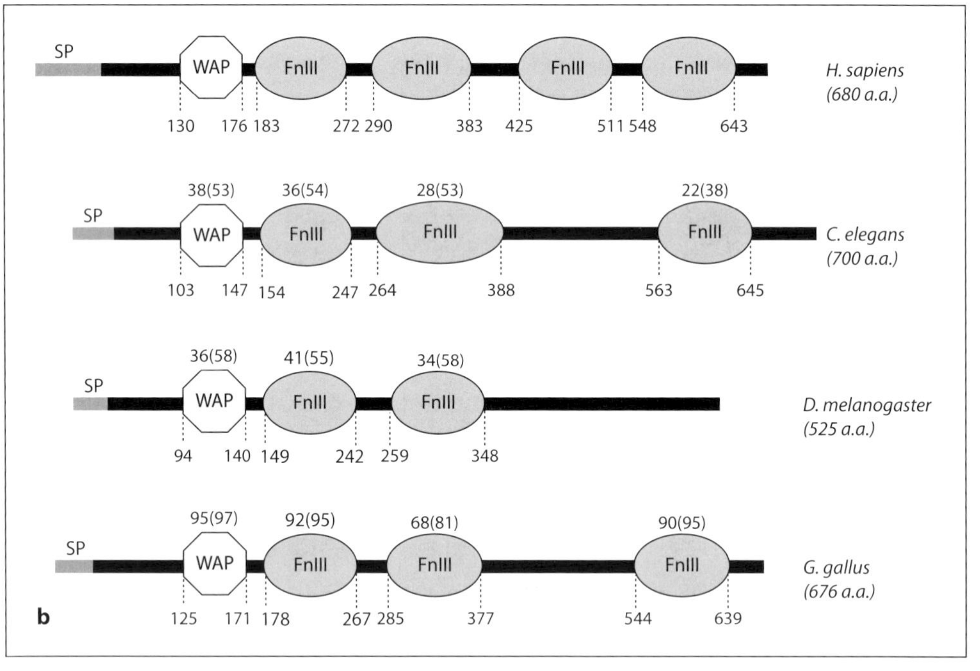

Fig. 1. **a** Structure of *KAL1* gene and anosmin-1 protein. Schematic representation of human *KAL1* cDNA and anosmin-1 protein. The *KAL1* gene is composed of 14 exons encoding a 2.4 kb of transcript and 680 amino acids. The six putative N-glycosylation sites and five potential HS binding sites are indicated and amino acid residues for each are shown. Nucleotide numbers for each exon are also shown. There is a signal peptide (SP) followed by a cysteine rich N-terminus (Cys Box), WAP-like four-disulphide core motif and four FnIII domains ending with a histidine (H)-rich C-terminus. The WAP domain and the first FnIII domain are functionally essential. Anosmin-1 lacks a transmembrane anchorage, thus is likely to be ECM-associated and secreted. **b** Conservation of functional domains of anosmin-1 through evolution. The domain structures of the anosmin-1 proteins based on SMART (http://smart.embl-heidelberg.de/smart). *Homo sapiens* (sequence ID:P23352), *C. elegans* (sequence ID: Q8WS94), *D. melanogaster* (sequence ID: Q9VCC7) and *Gallus gallus* (sequence ID: UPI000012DC04) are aligned. The relative positions of each domain in amino acid residues are shown as the numbers below the dotted lines. The numbers above each domain represent the percentage of identities and positives (shown in parentheses) compared to human, which is determined by alignment of the corresponding protein sequences of each domain using BLAST (www.ncbi.nlm.nih.gov/blast).

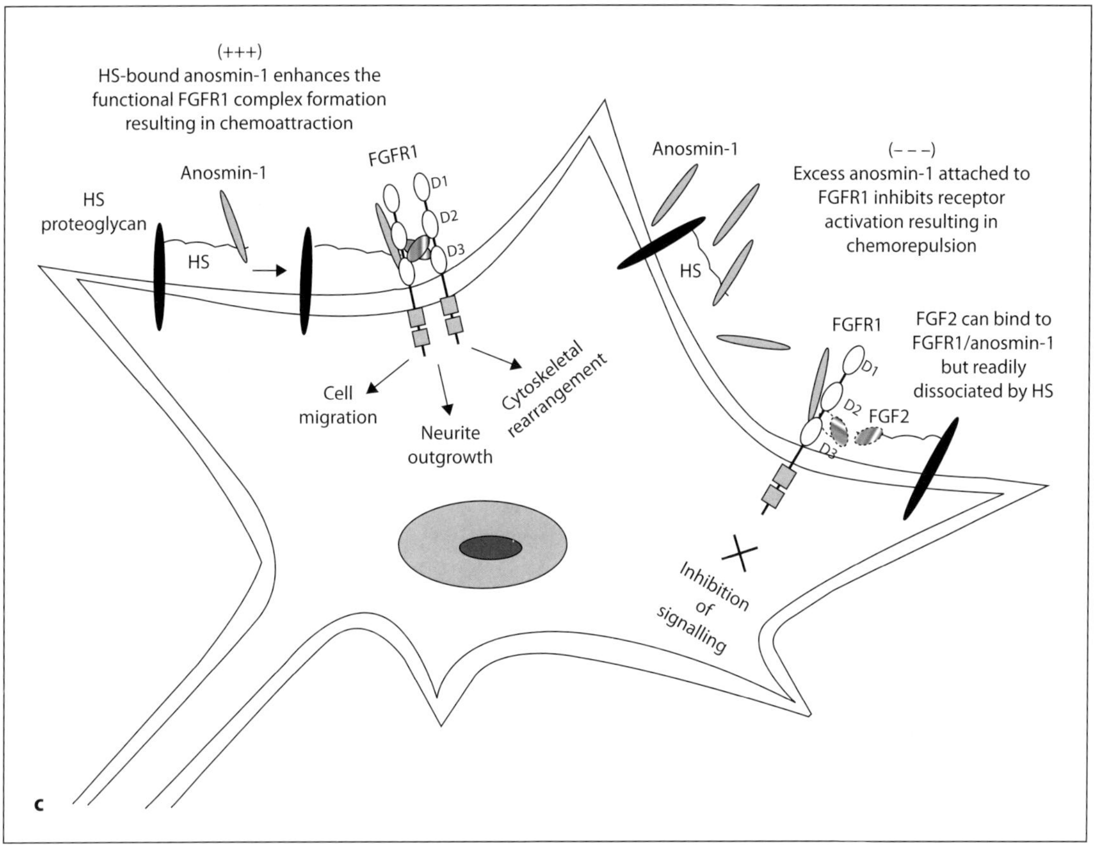

Fig. 1. **c** Putative mechanisms of molecular interaction between anosmin-1, FGFR1, FGF2 and HS on the cell surface. When HS-bound anosmin-1 associates with an otherwise transient complex between FGFR1 and FGF2, a stable anosmin-1/FGFR1/FGF2/HS complex forms leading to activation of the receptor and the consequent network of FGFR1 signalling pathways as indicated. On the other hand, when there is high-level expression of anosmin-1 potentially exceeding the binding capacity of the local HS, free anosmin-1 attaches with high affinity to FGFR1, preventing the formation of an FGF2/FGFR1/HS signalling complex.

elastin [18]. HE4 is a serological tumour biomarker used to predict ovarian cancer and has a presumptive role in natural immunity [19]. WDNM1 is an extracellular proteinase inhibitor whose downregulation has been linked with metastatic rat mammary adenocarcinomas [20]. Finally, ps20 has protease-inhibitory activity and can stimulate endothelial cell migration and promotes angiogenesis and tumour growth in a prostate cancer model [21], though in a different study, ps20 was shown to inhibit the proliferation of prostate carcinoma cells [22]. In all, WAP family of proteins exhibit protease inhibitory activity, regulate cell proliferation, differentiation and tissue remodelling in various tissue types. That the WAP domain is evolutionarily conserved in all anosmin-1 sequences suggests that anosmin-1 might also be capable of some of these functions. However, it has been shown that anosmin-1 promoted, rather than inhibited, the proteolytic activities of urokinase type plasminogen activator (uPA) in vitro, while exogenous addition of anosmin-1 induced cell proliferation in prostate carcinoma cell line PC3 [13]. The activity of the WAP domain might be affected in the C172R or C163Y missense mutations found in KS patients, since these substitutions are thought to disrupt the conserved C151–C163, C157–C172 disulphide bonds, probably affecting the protein folding or structural stability of this region.

D. melanogaster has two, chicken and *C. elegans* have three and human has four FnIII domains in anosmin-1 protein (fig. 1b). The FnIII domains of anosmin-1 have significant homology with members of the cell adhesion molecule (CAM) family including fibronectin, neural CAM (NCAM), L1 and tenasin. These molecules are usually associated with extracellular and cell-cell interaction, adhesion, proliferation and migration during neuronal development, suggesting a similar involvement of anosmin-1 in these cellular processes. FnIII is a small autonomous folding unit which occurs in many proteins involved in ligand binding and dimerisation [23], and it has been shown that FnIII domains in NCAM, L1, N-Cadherin, Sef and *Xenopus* fibronectin leucine-rich transmembrane protein 3 (XFLRT3) play essential roles in their binding interactions with FGFR1 [24–28]. Consistently, our recent study demonstrated that anosmin-1 directly binds to FGFR1 through the FnIII domain [17]. Since the arrangement of the six domains of anosmin-1 in solution state appears extended, with flexible inter-domain linkers, it has been speculated that anosmin-1 may interact with multiple molecules providing a binding platform or scaffolding for potential multiprotein complex formation on the cell surface [29]. There are five putative heparan sulphate (HS) binding sites amongst or within the individual FnIII domains of anosmin-1 (fig. 1a). HS-mediated cell surface association is essential for anosmin-1's activity [30, 31]. HS acts as a receptor or co-receptor to regulate the biological activities of HS-binding proteins to promote dimerisation of its ligand and receptor, induce receptor phosphorylation and stabilise an active ligand-receptor complex formation. Interaction studies between the HS and FGF system is one of the best studied examples [32] and will be discussed further in relation to anosmin-1 in the later section. The predominant loss-of-function mutations (frameshift, deletions) with 10 missense mutations are identified in the WAP and the first FnIII domains so far and five missense mutations identified have been mapped closely to the putative HS binding sites. It is speculated that N267K (in first FnIII domain) and E514K (in third FnIII domain) mutations associated with X-KS cases may enhance HS binding as these are neutral/negative to positive amino acid substitutions and the increased HS binding may inhibit the molecular movement or flexibility of anosmin-1 in the ECM. An F517L substitution (in third FnIII domain), although occurs close to an HS binding domain, does not change the charge of amino acids; thus, it is not clear how this mutation affects the activity of anosmin-1. The correlation of individual domains of anosmin-1 contributing to different biological activities will be discussed further in detail later.

Expression of *KAL1* and Anosmin-1 during Human Development

The degree of hypogonadism and anosmia in KS patients can vary significantly within the pedigree [33], even between monozygotic twins [34]. Despite this considerable phenotypic variability within and between KS kindreds, the phenotype associated with *KAL1* mutations is fairly constant, with renal aplasia and bimanual synkinesis being far more prevalent in X-KS (albeit no longer thought to be specific markers) at up to 30% and 75% of cases, respectively [35]. Thus, anosmin-1 may have specific roles during the organogenesis of kidney and upper motor neuron development, in addition to its presumed roles in cranial nerve I complex axon guidance, GnRH neuron migration and OB morphogenesis.

Investigation of the expression patterns of *KAL1* gene and anosmin-1 protein during embryonic development has produced results coinciding with the clinical phenotypes and forms a good basis to further contemplate the biological roles of anosmin-1 and the potential pathways that it governs. Anosmin-1 expression was detected from a 5-week-old human embryo in the interstitial matrix of the presumptive OB before the first contact that the olfactory axons make with the telecephalon [14]. Anosmin-1 was also detected in the nasal placode at 4.5 weeks, alongside the terminal nerve at 8 weeks and in the medial wall of the primitive cerebral hemispheres along the pathways of the GnRH neuronal migration and their associated nerve fibres at 6 weeks of human development [14]. Furthermore, *KAL1* mRNA was shown to be present in the olfactory nerve layer and granular cell layer of the OB at 19 weeks [2]. Based on these findings, it has been proposed that anosmin-1 is a short-range neuronal guidance molecule that aids the olfactory axonal trajectory and may also play a direct role during the OB differentiation. Loss-of-function mutations of anosmin-1, as found in X-linked KS patients, would disrupt the olfactory nerve synaptogenesis with the primordial OB, which in turn results in critical hypothalamic GnRH neuronal deficiency since the late wave of GnRH neuronal migration towards the forebrain follows this olfactory axonal migratory route. Anosmin-1 detection in the mesonephric duct and uretic bud branches from week 5 onwards suggests a direct involvement of anosmin-1 during early nephrogenesis, whose defects may be responsible for renal aplasis in X-KS cases. The anosmin-1 protein is also expressed in the otic vesicle and its derivatives, corresponding with the sensorineural hearing defects found in some KS cases [14].

Studies of *KAL1*/anosmin-1 expression in embryos of different animals have provided results in line with the findings from human fetal tissues, and yet also revealed some differences, which suggest that careful distinction and validation of these characteristics will be necessary before they are used as the KS disease models. Conversely, any new findings from animal studies may trigger re-examination of human subjects for any subtle characteristics which may have been overlooked in earlier human studies. For instance, in chicken, high levels of *kal-1* transcript were similarly found in the OB mitral neurons that form synapses with olfactory axons as well as in the cerebellar purkinje cells, retinal neurons and some neuronal populations of the brainstem and spinal cord, agreeing that anosmin-1 is a signal molecule required for neuronal targeting. In contrast, low or no levels were observed in the developing kidney, olfactory epithelium or the surrounding nasal mesenchyme [37].

Functions of Anosmin-1

The biological roles of anosmin-1 have been investigated by independent groups over the years using various cellular and biochemical systems. Anosmin-1 exhibits activities in cell adhesion, migration, axon guidance/branching, neurite outgrowth and cell proliferation, as well as differential roles in head skeleton/wing formation in fly and lateral line establishment/hearing in fish [12–14, 16, 30, 38–47].

The potential function of anosmin-1 as an adhesion molecule has been reported in neuronal and non-neuronal cells, although the underlying molecular mechanism is still not clear [31, 42, 43]. Co-culture experiments have shown that anosmin-1 can promote neurite outgrowth. Five-day-old (P5) mouse cerebellar neurons developed longer neurites when cultured on wells coated with anosmin-1, whereas anosmin-1 had no effect on E18 hippocampal and P1 dorsal root ganglion neurons, suggesting these activities were cell type specific [44]. In rat OB explant organo-culture, anosmin-1 can stimulate lateral olfactory tract neurite branching and neuronal outgrowth from the mitral and tufted cells in the OB towards the pyriform cortex [45]. Since these olfactory collaterals are the sole connection between the OB and the cerebral cortex, loss of anosmin-1 function will cause defective olfaction even if normal OB morphogenesis has occurred. In fact, some X-KS individuals have compromised sense of smell despite the presence of apparently normal looking OB on MR imaging [48]. It has also been shown that anosmin-1 added exogenously to immortalized mouse GnRH neurons display specific chemotactic activity in culture [30]. Anosmin-1 produced a cell-specific chemotactic response of GN11, a subclone of GnRH secreting neuron cells, but not in GT1–7 cells, mature postmigratory mouse GnRH neuronal cells. However, none of the KS-associated missense mutations (N267K, E514K and F517L) of anosmin-1 affected this chemotactic activity in this study [30]. Anosmin-1 has also been previously reported to inhibit the migration of mouse oligodendrocyte precursor cells [42]. On the other hand, we have shown that addition of recombinant anosmin-1 protein at low concentrations can stimulate human GnRH neuroblasts FNC-B4 to induce neurite outgrowth [36] and Transwell migration [17], but inhibits these responses at high concentrations. In both situations, anosmin-1 effects were mediated via FGFR1- and HS-dependent mechanisms [17, 36]. These varying observations from different studies may reflect anosmin-1's potential to serve as either chemoattractant or chemorepellent in different cell types through its interaction with multiple cell surface molecules, which may also depend on their relative expression levels.

The mis-/overexpression of anosmin-1 has been used in two animal models providing further insights into the role of anosmin-1 in different contexts. Neuron-specific forced expression of *kal-1* in *C. elegans* caused axonal branching defects, although the overall functionality of the neurons seemed normal. Pan-neuronal expression of *kal-1* resulted in axon mis-routing as well as head and tail morphogenesis defects [31]. In this context, a CeKal-1 loss of function mutation as well as CeKal-1 overexpression similarly produced ventral closure and male tail defects. On the other hand, overexpression of DmKal-1 in *D. melanogaster* induced dose-dependent structural defects in the cephalopharyngeal skeleton and the wing disc [47]. Both studies attempted a structure-function dissection of the anosmin-1 protein to establish whether a particular domain(s) of anosmin-1 is responsible for a specific function(s), which will be further discussed later in this review.

Interactions of Anosmin-1 with Other Molecules

Heparan Sulphate Mediates Anosmin-1 Interactions on the Cell Surface

Anosmin-1 requires HS for its function. HS proteoglycans (HSPGs) are cell surface- and ECM-associated proteins with HS glycosaminoglycan side chains attached to the core protein. The HS are long carbohydrate chains composed of alternating disaccharide repeats of glucuronic acid or iduronic acid and glucosamine residues with variable sulphation patterns. The fine structure of the sulphation pattern is responsible for specific binding and regulatory functions of a number of HS-binding proteins, including growth factors and cytokines, mediating various normal and pathological cellular functions. Thus, the spatiotemporal HSPG expression and HS structural modification are precisely regulated [50]. Consistently, deletion of the major HS glycosyltransferase *Ext1* in mice is lethal at gastrulation and causes failure in mesoderm formation [51], and the cortical progenitor cells derived from these mice show no proliferative response to FGF2/FGF8 treatment [52].

The high affinity binding between anosmin-1 and HS has been confirmed by surface plasmon resonance analysis using purified recombinant anosmin-1 proteins, and the first FnIII domain was shown to contain the major HS-binding activity. Wild-type and WAP-mutated (C172R) full-length anosmin-1 have higher HS-binding affinity than the C-terminal truncated version missing the FnIII domains, indicating that the increasing numbers of FnIII domains allow stronger HS binding, and the WAP domain is not essential for HS interaction [13]. Interaction of anosmin-1 on the cell membrane is critically dependent on the presence of HS, and this can be blocked by addition of exogenous heparin or heparanase treatment [16, 30, 31]. To reinforce this notion, in vivo studies using transgenic *C. elegans* showed that worms lacking 6-O-sulphotransferase *(hst-6)* or *C5*-epimerase *(hse-5)* abolished the specific axon-branching phenotype induced by anosmin-1 but caused little effect in those lacking 2-O-sulphotransferase *(hst-2)* [31, 53], implying that these sulphation events may be relevant in exerting anosmin-1 action. It was also suggested that syndecan and glypican may be the cell surface HSPG core proteins which interact with anosmin-1 via an HS-dependent mechanism [54]. Although it is not yet known whether any of these sulphotransferases or HSPGs are potential KS genes, it is a highly plausible idea since, in addition to anosmin-1, other KS-associated proteins (FGFR1, FGF8, PROK2, PROKR2) also have HS-binding capacity and/or require HS for their activity, and could thus cooperate in converging signalling pathways mediated via HS interactions.

Anosmin-1 Interacts with Extracellular Protease uPA

uPA, a serine protease known to be expressed in the developing OB, spinal cord and kidney epithelial cells, is often expressed in areas of neuronal projections in early embryogenesis [55]. uPA activates plasmin, which then further initiates a range of protease systems on the cell surface to release activated growth factors and degrade ECM components, which are essential for cell migration, invasion, tissue re-modelling and angiogenesis. It was shown that anosmin-1 directly binds to uPA and significantly enhances the proteolytic activity of uPA in vitro in a dose-dependent manner, but showed no effect on thrombin, indicating that anosmin-1 effect may be specific. Anosmin-1 induces cell proliferation in a prostate cancer cell line (PC-3) in an HS-dependent manner and the WAP domain is required for this activity [13]. Increased uPA activity can lead to activation and release of several growth factors such as insulin-like growth factor and FGF. However, whether the observed mitogenic capacity of anosmin-1 is dependent on uPA-mediated proteolysis or involves uPA receptor signalling pathway is unknown. uPA is also an HS-binding protein, thus HS could concentrate and restrict the distribution of uPA/anosmin-1 on the cell surface.

Anosmin-1 Modulates the FGFR1 Signalling Pathway

After the initial identification of overlapping interstitial deletions at 8p11-p12 in 2 individuals with contiguous gene syndromes, germline mutations of FGFR1 are recognized as the underlying genetic defects *(KAL2)* for the autosomal dominant (with highly variable penetrance) form of KS [7]. FGFR1 belongs to the FGFR receptor tyrosine kinase family whose signalling pathways play fundamental roles during cell proliferation, migration, survival and differentiation, thus involved in a range of physiological and pathological processes such as development, repair, homeostasis and tumourigenesis. Like other FGFRs, FGFR1 consists of an extracellular ligand binding domain, a single transmembrane domain and a cytoplasmic kinase domain. The extracellular domain contains three immunoglobulin-like domains named D1, D2 and D3. The D2-D3 contains FGF- and HS-binding sites. The dimerisation of FGFR1 is initiated by binding of ligand FGFs. However, HS is required to stabilise this relatively weak binding between FGFR and FGF and facilitate the signalling events. The details of FGFR1 biology, signalling mechanisms, and mutations contributing to KS phenotypes are discussed in other chapters of this volume.

Recent reports support the notion that anosmin-1 and FGFR1 are involved in the same cellular signalling pathway and in fact, anosmin-1 is an extracellular regulator of FGFR1. These include the study on FNC-B4 cells derived from human fetal olfactory epithelium, which express several olfactory and neuron specific markers as well as GnRH-1 and GnRH receptor and respond to autocrine GnRH stimulation. Adding recombinant anosmin-1 protein to these cells induced neurite outgrowth and actin cytoskeletal rearrangement through FGFR1/FGF2-mediated signalling pathways which induced sustained phosphorylation of MAP kinases (p42/p44 and p38, but not JNK), accompanied by Cdc42/Rac1 activation. This effect seemed to be through physical interaction with FGFR1/FGF2/HSPG complex on the cell surface, which could be co-immunoprecipitated with anosmin-1. In BaF3 cell system expressing an individual FGFR isoform, anosmin-1 showed specific activity on FGFR1 IIIc isoform in an HS-dependent manner [36]. Anosmin-1 may also interact with FGFR1 to modulate FGF2-dependent events in the developing optic nerve. In this study, the mouse oligodendrocyte precursor cells migrate out of the optic nerve explants upon addition of FGF2. Anosmin-1 did not show any chemotropic or chemotactic effects in this system, but significantly reduced the number of cells migrating. This phenomenon also seems to be mediated by FGFR1/anosmin-1 interaction since addition of soluble FGFR1 IIIc recombinant protein resulted in reversal of the anosmin-1 effect and the FGFR1/anosmin-1 complex could be co-immunoprecipitated from the membrane fraction isolated from the E15 brain [42].

Currently, there are several proteins in addition to anosmin-1 that have been shown to modulate FGFR signalling, some of which show direct protein-protein interaction with FGFR1; Sprouty protein family and the related protein, Spred, inhibit FGFR signalling and FGFR-mediated cell motility through attenuation of the downstream Ras-ERK pathway; Sef (similar expression to fgf genes) functions as an antagonist of FGF signalling in zebrafish and has two extracellular FnIII regions [26]; XFLRT3 is a transmembrane protein with an extracellular FnIII domain, which promotes FGFR signalling [24]; NCAM is structurally and functionally related to anosmin-1, showing FGFR-mediated neurite outgrowth, but unlike anosmin-1, it can induce ligand-independent activation of FGFR1 [27]. These findings strongly imply that there are additional levels of FGFR signal regulation other than the conventional ligands and their pairing with different FGFR isoforms and HSPG co-receptors.

Domain-Specific Interactions between Anosmin-1 and FGFR1

Although anosmin-1 was shown to co-immunoprecipitate with the FGF2/FGFR1/HS complex [36, 42], the exact molecular interactions within the multiprotein complex had not been completely elucidated. Our recent study showed that anosmin-1 directly binds to FGFR1 with high affinity, and this occurs between the N-terminus of anosmin-1 (cysteine-rich region, WAP and the first FnIII domain) and the D2-D3 domains of FGFR1 [17]. The major FGFR1 binding site is likely to be located in the first FnIII domain because the C-terminal truncated anosmin-1 containing only the first FnIII domain retains the FGFR1 binding capacity, but a point mutation N267K in the first FnIII domain results in complete loss of binding, while mutations in the third FnIII domain do not. However, the cysteine-rich and WAP domains are still required for the interaction since the four FnIII domains alone cannot bind to FGFR1. It was also demonstrated that anosmin-1 binds to FGFR2IIIc with much lower affinity and has little affinity for FGFR3IIIc, making a preferential binding order of FGFR1>FGFR2>FGFR3; this finding is consistent with our previous observation from the BaF3 cell system where anosmin-1 has effects only on cells expressing FGFR1IIIc, but not FGFR2IIIc and FGFR3IIIc isoforms. Furthermore, using a serial injection technique in surface plasmon resonance experiments, it is shown that HS-bound anosmin-1 binds to pre-formed FGF2/FGFR1 complex, resulting in anosmin-1/FGFR1/FGF2/HS complex. This result supports a scenario where anosmin-1 may 'present' or 'recruit' the appropriate HS to the FGFR1/FGF2 complex that would otherwise just be a transient binding interaction. Thus, anosmin-1 could promote the formation of a stable and functional signalling complex. On the other hand, the data also show that when anosmin-1 is bound to FGFR1 first, the FGFR1/anosmin-1 heterodimer cannot bind to pre-formed FGF2/HS complex, thus preventing functional FGFR1/FGF2/HS signalling complex formation. In this scenario, anosmin-1 may function instead as an antagonist of FGFR1 signalling activity (fig. 1c) [17].

In some respects, these results should not be surprising, since several molecules that are known to regulate and interact with FGFR, such as NCAM, N-cadherin, L1, Sef and XFLRT3, have all shown direct protein-protein binding via their extracellular FnIII domains, indicating that there could be a common molecular motif involved in these interactions. Nevertheless, it appears that these proteins use different molecular mechanisms, and that domains other than FnIII also play important roles in delivering the biological activity. For example, NCAM may induce co-clustering of the FGFR by homophilic binding, leading to ligand-independent receptor activation [56]. XFLRT3 binds with FGFR1 and FGFR4 directly through its extracellular FnIII domain, but the ability to promote FGF signalling is dependent on the cytoplasmic tail [24]. Unlike other FGFR1-binding proteins, however, anosmin-1 is a secretory molecule which can diffuse forming a concentration gradient potentially regulating biological responses of the target cells. The HSPGs anchored on the plasma membrane may be able to restrict anosmin-1 diffusion and the HS-bound anosmin-1 will preferentially associate with pre-existing FGF/FGFR complex to facilitate FGF/FGFR/HS signalling activity. When anosmin-1 is highly expressed, in excess of the binding capacity of the cell surface HS, however, the free anosmin-1 would attach to FGFR1, resulting in inhibition of FGFR1 signalling complex formation. The opposing effects of anosmin-1 on FGFR1 as seen in this study provide new evidence that anosmin-1 may be a guidance molecule with both attractive and repelling properties which, in cooperation with FGFR1 downstream effectors, directs cell migration and axon pathfinding during GnRH neuronal migration and neurite outgrowth. The relative binding capacity and specific structure of HS on the cell surface and the expression levels of anosmin-1 within the local cellular environment at a particular developmental stage may shift anosmin-1 either into a FGFR1-bound or HS-bound state, consequently determining the biological outcome. Therefore, it can be envisaged that agents that affect anosmin-1's affinity with FGFR1 or HS may be potentially used as pharmacological tools to modulate FGFR1 signalling activity.

Structure-Function Relationship of Anosmin-1

The highest conservation of sequences in anosmin-1 is confined within the N-terminal WAP and first FnIII domain (fig. 1b), so these two domains are likely to be functionally important. Independent groups attempted to dissect the distinct domains of anosmin-1 in terms of specific contribution toward their biological activities. For instance, in *C. elegans*, the WAP domain influences the misrouting and axon targeting phenotype, whilst the FnIII domains are required for neurite outgrowth and axon branching, although both are still dependent on HS interactions. The N267K-equivalent mutation in the first FnIII domain abolished HS-dependent cell adhesion and axonal branching in *C. elegans* [31], similar to the human counterpart which caused loss of the migration activity on GN11 cells [30]. In contrast, the equivalent substitution in *Drosophila* did not alter anosmin-1 interaction on the cell surface. It has been speculated that this might be due to the fact that a conserved HS binding site (XBBXBX where X is a random and B is a basic residue) located near to the site of the N267K mutation is not present in *Drosophila*. In the context of the wing development, however, the N267K equivalent substitution did cause loss of the DmKal-1-induced phenotype, but the WAP domain was dispensable in this context [47]. WAP mutation of *C. elegans kal-1* abrogated the HS-dependent binding activity [31], while the similar mutation in human did not affect the HS-binding potential [13]. This apparent discrepancy may be due to the intrinsic differences of the ECM composition in different species, and the fact that WAP domain is not essential in some cell context may explain the case of an X-KS patient with the C163Y mutation in the WAP domain, who only had a relatively mild phenotype [57]. The functional interdependence between the WAP and FnIII repeats has been demonstrated previously; the phenotype induced by overexpression of the N267K-equivalent mutant in *Drosophila* was suppressed by the mutation of WAP domain [47]. Moreover, we have previously reported that C-terminal truncated anosmin-1 containing only the first FnIII domain is sufficient to induce neurite outgrowth in the FNC-B4 cells in culture, but a point mutation in the WAP domain (C172R) abolishes this activity [36]. These data suggest that the function of the WAP domain is somehow linked to the function of the FnIII domain, and it is plausible that the WAP domain and possibly the cysteine-rich region regulate or support FnIII to conform the appropriate orientation.

Discussion and Conclusions

Since anosmin-1 was first identified as a KS-associated protein, an increasing number of studies have suggested that it has multiple biological roles. It is highly likely that anosmin-1 has several interacting partners, depending on the cell context determining the differential responses to FGF and other signalling cues, whose deficiency is attributed to the KS phenotypes. Such examples would include its interaction with HS, FGFR1 and uPA, and this list may further expand in the future. The functions of anosmin-1 may be mediated by cognate receptors with which it has direct or indirect interactions and whose activation leads to various intracellular signalling events.

It was originally proposed that anosmin-1 was a neuronal guidance molecule that determined the trajectory of ingrowing axons of the cranial nerve I complex [45]. Thus, loss of anosmin-1 function would disrupt the olfactory nerve synaptogenesis with the OB anlage, which then secondarily disrupts GnRH neuron migration towards the hypothalamus. However, a later study in *C. elegans* suggested that the olfactory targeting defect observed in X-KS might not necessarily result from loss of attraction of olfactory axons, but was rather an indirect consequence of misrouting of neurons within the OB which then renders them incapable of attracting/recognising the olfactory axons so as to allow correct innervation [31]. More recent studies using fish and fly models further support the notion that anosmin-1 can have a more general role in cell migration, including axon guidance, neuronal branching and morphogenesis [39, 46, 47, 49]. In any case, the HSPG is likely to be involved in mediating anosmin-1 action on the cell surface. Our recent report suggests that HS-bound anosmin-1 contributes to the formation of a functional signalling complex to the otherwise unstable FGFR1/FGF2 complexes. Whether anosmin-1's role in this scenario is to bring in the 'right' species of HS to the FGFR1 complex to warrant an efficient signalling activity has yet to be confirmed. Notably, 6-O-sulphation has been shown to be necessary for the function of both FGFR1 and anosmin-1. Conversely, it is also possible that anosmin-1 may aid FGFR1 to overcome the specific requirement of HS fine structure, thus allowing signalling events to occur in certain 'less-than-perfect' extracellular environments. The relative balance between the cell surface HS and anosmin-1 seems to be the key factor determining the outcome of anosmin-1 action. Further knowledge on specific HS structures that interact with anosmin-1 may help in answering these questions.

That hypogonadism and anosmia can occur separately in non-X-linked KS kindreds suggests that OB development may not always be directly linked to GnRH development [33, 35]. Bearing in mind that X-KS patients often display additional symptoms including synkinesis and unilateral renal agenesis, other functions of anosmin-1 contributing to these phenotypes may well exist. Unveiling the novel functions and interactants of anosmin-1 and the signalling networks involved will provide exciting prospects and paves the way forward in understanding the molecular pathogenesis of KS.

References

1 Fromantin M, Grieste J, Didier A, Ronnier J: Les impuberisms et ls hypogonadisms a l'incorporation. Prob Actuels Endocrinol Nutr 1972;16:179–199.

2 Schwanzel-Fukuda M, Bick D, Pfaff DW: Luteinizing hormone-releasing hormone (LHRH)-expressing cells do not migrate normally in an inherited hypogonadal (Kallmann) syndrome. Brain Res Mol Brain Res 1989;6:311–326.

3 Oliveira LM, Seminara SB, Beranova M, Hayes FJ, Valkenburgh SB, Schipani E, Costa EM, Latronico AC, Crowley WF Jr, Vallejo M: The importance of autosomal genes in Kallmann syndrome: genotype-phenotype correlations and neuroendocrine characteristics. J Clin Endocrinol Metab 2001;86: 1532–1538.

4 Pitteloud N, Quinton R, Pearce S, et al: Digenic mutations account for variable phenotypes in idiopathic hypogonadotropic hypogonadism. J Clin Invest 2007;117:457–463.

5 Franco B, Guioli S, Pragliola A, Incerti B, Bardoni B, Tonlorenzi R, Carrozzo R, Maestrini E, Pieretti M, Taillon-Miller P, Brown CJ, Willard HF, Lawrence C, Persico MG, Camerino G, Ballabio A: A gene deleted in Kallmann's syndrome shares homology with neural cell adhesion and axonal path-finding molecules. Nature 1991;353:529–536.

6 Legouis R, Hardelin JP, Levilliers J, Claverie JM, Compain S, Wunderle V, Millasseau P, Le Paslier D, Cohen D, Caterina D, Bougueleret L, Delemarre-Van de Waal, Lutfalla G, Wessenbach J, Petit C: The candidate gene for the X-linked Kallmann syndrome encodes a protein related to adhesion molecules. Cell 1991;67:423–435.

7 Dode C, Levilliers J, Dupont JM, et al: Loss-of-function mutations in FGFR1 cause autosomal dominant Kallmann syndrome. Nat Genet 2003;33: 463–465.

8 Dode C, Teixeira L, Levilliers J, et al: Kallmann syndrome: mutations in the genes encoding prokineticin-2 and prokineticin receptor-2. PLoS Genet 2006; 2:e175.

9 Kim HG, Kurth I, Lan F, Meliciani I, Wenzel W, Eom SH, Kang GB, Rosenberger G, Tekin M, Ozata M, Bick DP, Sherins RJ, Walker SL, Shi Y, Gusella JF, Layman LC: Mutations in CHD7, encoding a chromatin-remodeling protein, cause idiopathic hypogonadotropic hypogonadism and Kallmann syndrome. Am J Hum Genet 2008;83:511–519.

10 Falardeau J, Chung WC, Beenken A, et al: Decreased FGF8 signaling causes deficiency of gonadotropin-releasing hormone in humans and mice. J Clin Invest 2008;118:2822–2831.

11 Kim SH, Hu Y, Cadman S, Bouloux P: Diversity in fibroblast growth factor receptor 1 regulation: learning from the investigation of Kallmann syndrome. J Neuroendocrinol 2008;20:141–163.

12 Rugarli EI, Ghezzi C, Valsecchi V, Ballabio A: The Kallmann syndrome gene product expressed in COS cells is cleaved on the cell surface to yield a diffusible component. Hum Mol Genet 1996;5:1109–1115.

13 Hu Y, Gonzalez-Martinez D, Kim SH, Bouloux PM: Cross-talk of anosmin-1, the protein implicated in X-linked Kallmann's syndrome, with heparan sulphate and urokinase-type plasminogen activator. Biochem J 2004;384:495–505.

14 Hardelin JP, Julliard AK, Moniot B, Soussi-Yanicostas N, Verney C, Schwanzel-Fukuda M, Ayer-Le Lievre C, Petit C: Anosmin-1 is a regionally restricted component of basement membranes and interstitial matrices during organogenesis: implications for the developmental anomalies of X chromosome-linked Kallmann syndrome. Dev Dyn 1999; 215:26–44.

15 Zhao YY, Takahashi M, Gu JG, Miyoshi E, Matsumoto A, Kitazume S, Taniguchi N: Functional roles of N-glycans in cell signaling and cell adhesion in cancer. Cancer Sci 2008;99:1304–1310.

16 Soussi-Yanicostas N, Hardelin JP, Arroyo-Jimenez MM, Ardouin O, Legouis R, Levilliers J, Traincard F, Betton JM, Cabanie L, Petit C: Initial characterization of anosmin-1, a putative extracellular matrix protein synthesized by definite neuronal cell populations in the central nervous system. J Cell Sci 1996;109 (Pt 7):1749–1757.

17 Hu Y, Guimond SE, Travers P, Cadman SM, Hohenester E, Turnbull JE, Kim SH, Bouloux PM: Novel mechanism of fibroblast growth factor receptor 1 regulation by extracellular matrix protein anosmin-1. J Biol Chem 2009;284 :29905–29920.

18 King AE, Wheelhouse N, Cameron S, McDonald SE, Lee KF, Entrican G, Critchley HO, Horne AW: Expression of secretory leukocyte protease inhibitor and elafin in human fallopian tube and in an in-vitro model of Chlamydia trachomatis infection. Hum Reprod 2008;24:679–686.

19 Galgano MT, Hampton GM, Frierson HF Jr: Comprehensive analysis of HE4 expression in normal and malignant human tissues. Mod Pathol 2006;19: 847–853.

20 Dear TN, Kefford RF: The WDNM1 gene product is a novel member of the 'four-disulphide core' family of proteins. Biochem Biophys Res Commun 1991; 176:247–254.

21 Watson JE, Kamkar S, James K, Kowbel D, Andaya A, Paris PL, Simko J, Carroll P, McAlhany S, Rowley D, Collins C: Molecular analysis of WFDC1/ps20 gene in prostate cancer. Prostate 2004;61:192–199.

22 Larsen M, Ressler SJ, Lu B, Gerdes MJ, McBride L, Dang TD, Rowley DR: Molecular cloning and expression of ps20 growth inhibitor. A novel WAP-type 'four-disulfide core' domain protein expressed in smooth muscle. J Biol Chem 1998;273:4574–4584.

23 Koide A, Bailey CW, Huang X, Koide S: The fibronectin type III domain as a scaffold for novel binding proteins. J Mol Biol 1998;284:1141–1151.

24 Bottcher RT, Pollet N, Delius H, Niehrs C: The transmembrane protein XFLRT3 forms a complex with FGF receptors and promotes FGF signalling. Nat Cell Biol 2004;6:38–44.

25 Kulahin N, Li S, Hinsby A, Kiselyov V, Berezin V, Bock E: Fibronectin type III (FN3) modules of the neuronal cell adhesion molecule L1 interact directly with the fibroblast growth factor (FGF) receptor. Mol Cell Neurosci 2008;37:528–536.

26 Tsang M, Friesel R, Kudoh T, Dawid IB: Identification of Sef, a novel modulator of FGF signalling. Nat Cell Biol 2002;4:165–169.

27 Kiselyov VV, Skladchikova G, Hinsby AM, Jensen PH, Kulahin N, Soroka V, Pedersen N, Tsetlin V, Poulsen FM, Berezin V, Bock E: Structural basis for a direct interaction between FGFR1 and NCAM and evidence for a regulatory role of ATP. Structure 2003;11:691–701.

28 Williams EJ, Williams G, Howell FV, Skaper SD, Walsh FS, Doherty P: Identification of an N-cadherin motif that can interact with the fibroblast growth factor receptor and is required for axonal growth. J Biol Chem 2001;276:43879–43886.

29 Hu Y, Sun Z, Eaton JT, Bouloux PM, Perkins SJ: Extended and flexible domain solution structure of the extracellular matrix protein anosmin-1 by X-ray scattering, analytical ultracentrifugation and constrained modelling. J Mol Biol 2005;350:553–570.

30 Cariboni A, Pimpinelli F, Colamarino S, Zaninetti R, Piccolella M, Rumio C, Piva F, Rugarli EI, Maggi R: The product of X-linked Kallmann's syndrome gene (KAL1) affects the migratory activity of gonadotropin-releasing hormone (GnRH)-producing neurons. Hum Mol Genet 2004;13:2781–2791.

31 Bülow HE, Berry KL, Topper LH, Peles E, Hobert O: Heparan sulfate proteoglycan-dependent induction of axon branching and axon misrouting by the Kallmann syndrome gene kal-1. Proc Natl Acad Sci USA 2002;99:6346–6351.

32 Guimond SE, Turnbull JE: Fibroblast growth factor receptor signalling is dictated by specific heparan sulphate saccharides. Curr Biol 1999;9:1343–1346.

33 Pitteloud N, Hayes FJ, Boepple PA, DeCruz S, Seminara SB, MacLaughlin DT, Crowley WF Jr: The role of prior pubertal development, biochemical markers of testicular maturation, and genetics in elucidating the phenotypic heterogeneity of idiopathic hypogonadotropic hypogonadism. J Clin Endocrinol Metab 2002;87:152–160.

34 Hipkin LJ, Casson IF, Davis JC: Identical twins discordant for Kallmann's syndrome. J Med Genet 1990;27:198–199.

35 Quinton R, Duke VM, Robertson A, Kirk JM, Matfin G, de Zoysa PA, Azcona C, MacColl GS, Jacobs HS, Conway GS, Besser M, Stanhope RG, Bouloux PM: Idiopathic gonadotrophin deficiency: genetic questions addressed through phenotypic characterization. Clin Endocrinol (Oxf) 2001;55: 163–174.

36 Gonzalez-Martinez D, Kim SH, Hu Y, Guimond S, Schofield J, Winyard P, Vannelli GB, Turnbull J, Bouloux PM: Anosmin-1 modulates fibroblast growth factor receptor 1 signaling in human gonadotropin-releasing hormone olfactory neuroblasts through a heparan sulfate-dependent mechanism. J Neurosci 2004;24:10384–10392.

37 Lutz B, Kuratani S, Rugarli EI, Wawersik S, Wong C, Bieber FR, Ballabio A, Eichele G: Expression of the Kallmann syndrome gene in human fetal brain and in the manipulated chick embryo. Hum Mol Genet 1994;3:1717–1723.

38 Ardouin O, Legouis R, Fasano L, David-Watine B, Korn H, Hardelin J, Petit C: Characterization of the two zebrafish orthologues of the KAL-1 gene underlying X chromosome-linked Kallmann syndrome. Mech Dev 2000;90:89–94.

39 Okubo K, Sakai F, Lau EL, Yoshizaki G, Takeuchi Y, Naruse K, Aida K, Nagahama Y: Forebrain gonadotropin-releasing hormone neuronal development: insights from transgenic medaka and the relevance to X-linked Kallmann syndrome. Endocrinology 2006;147:1076–1084.

40 Ernest S, Guadagnini S, Prevost MC, Soussi-Yanicostas N: Localization of anosmin-1a and anosmin-1b in the inner ear and neuromasts of zebrafish. Gene Expr Patterns 2007;7:274–281.

41 Andrenacci D, Le Bras S, Rosaria GM, Rugarli E, Graziani F: Embryonic expression pattern of the Drosophila Kallmann syndrome gene kal-1. Gene Expr Patterns 2004;5:67–73.

42 Bribian A, Barallobre MJ, Soussi-Yanicostas N, de Castro F: Anosmin-1 modulates the FGF-2-dependent migration of oligodendrocyte precursors in the developing optic nerve. Mol Cell Neurosci 2006;33: 2–14.

43 Robertson A, MacColl GS, Nash JA, Boehm MK, Perkins SJ, Bouloux PM: Molecular modelling and experimental studies of mutation and cell-adhesion sites in the fibronectin type III and whey acidic protein domains of human anosmin-1. Biochem J 2001; 357:647–659.
44 Soussi-Yanicostas N, Faivre-Sarrailh C, Hardelin JP, Levilliers J, Rougon G, Petit C: Anosmin-1 underlying the X chromosome-linked Kallmann syndrome is an adhesion molecule that can modulate neurite growth in a cell-type specific manner. J Cell Sci 1998;111:2953–2965.
45 Soussi-Yanicostas N, de Castro F, Julliard AK, Perfettini I, Chedotal A, Petit C: Anosmin-1, defective in the X-linked form of Kallmann syndrome, promotes axonal branch formation from olfactory bulb output neurons. Cell 2002;109:217–228.
46 Yanicostas C, Ernest S, Dayraud C, Petit C, Soussi-Yanicostas N: Essential requirement for zebrafish anosmin-1a in the migration of the posterior lateral line primordium. Dev Biol 2008;320:469–479.
47 Andrenacci D, Grimaldi MR, Panetta V, Riano E, Rugarli EI, Graziani F: Functional dissection of the Drosophila Kallmann's syndrome protein DmKal-1. BMC Genet 2006;7:47–61.
48 Quinton R, Duke VM, de Zoysa PA, Platts AD, Valentine A, Kendall B, Pickman S, Kirk JM, Besser GM, Jacobs HS, Bouloux PM: The neuroradiology of Kallmann's syndrome: a genotypic and phenotypic analysis. J Clin Endocrinol Metab 1996;81: 3010–3017.
49 Whitlock KE, Smith KM, Kim H, Harden MV: A role for foxd3 and sox10 in the differentiation of gonadotropin-releasing hormone (GnRH) cells in the zebrafish *Danio rerio*. Development 2005;132: 5491–5502.
50 Brickman YG, Ford MD, Gallagher JT, Nurcombe V, Bartlett PF, Turnbull JE: Structural modification of fibroblast growth factor-binding heparan sulfate at a determinative stage of neural development. J Biol Chem 1998;273:4350–4359.
51 Lin X, Wei G, Shi Z, Dryer L, Esko JD, Wells DE, Matzuk MM: Disruption of gastrulation and heparan sulfate biosynthesis in EXT1-deficient mice. Dev Biol 2000;224:299–311.
52 Inatani M, Irie F, Plump AS, Tessier-Lavigne M, Yamaguchi Y: Mammalian brain morphogenesis and midline axon guidance require heparan sulfate. Science 2003;302:1044–1046.
53 Bülow HE, Hobert O: Differential sulfations and epimerization define heparan sulfate specificity in nervous system development. Neuron 2004;41:723–736.
54 Hudson ML, Kinnunen T, Cinar HN, Chisholm AD: C. elegans Kallmann syndrome protein KAL-1 interacts with syndecan and glypican to regulate neuronal cell migrations. Dev Biol 2006;294:352–365.
55 Dent MA, Sumi Y, Morris RJ, Seeley PJ: Urokinase-type plasminogen activator expression by neurons and oligodendrocytes during process outgrowth in developing rat brain. Eur J Neurosci 1993;5:633–647.
56 Doherty P, Williams G, Williams EJ: CAMs and axonal growth: a critical evaluation of the role of calcium and the MAPK cascade. Mol Cell Neurosci 2000;16:283–295.
57 Sato N, Katsumata N, Kagami M, et al: Clinical assessment and mutation analysis of Kallmann syndrome 1 (KAL1) and fibroblast growth factor receptor 1 (FGFR1, or KAL2) in five families and 18 sporadic patients. J Clin Endocrinol Metab 2004; 89:1079–1088.

Soo-Hyun Kim, PhD
Senior Lecturer
Division of Basic Medical Sciences, St. George's Medical School, University of London
Cranmer Terrace
London SW17 0RE (UK)
Tel. +44 20 82666198, Fax +44 20 87253326, E-Mail skim@sgul.ac.uk

Quinton R (ed): Kallmann Syndrome and Hypogonadotropic Hypogonadism.
Front Horm Res. Basel, Karger, 2010, vol 39, pp 94–110

Genotype and Phenotype of Patients with Gonadotropin-Releasing Hormone Receptor Mutations

Hyung-Goo Kim[a,b] · Jennifer Pedersen-White[c] · Balasubramanian Bhagavath[d] · Lawrence C. Layman[a,b]

[a]Section of Reproductive Endocrinology, Infertility, and Genetics, Department of Obstetrics and Gynecology, [b]Reproductive Medicine Program and Neurodevelopmental Biology Program, Institute of Molecular Medicine and Genetics, Neuroscience Program, and [c]Section of Endocrinology, Department of Medicine, Medical College of Georgia, Augusta, Ga., [d]Division of Reproductive Endocrinology and Infertility, Women and Infants' Hospital of Rhode Island, Brown University, Providence, R.I., USA

Abstract

Human mutations in the gonadotropin-releasing hormone receptor (*GNRHR*) gene cause autosomal recessive, normosmic idiopathic hypogonadotropic hypogonadism (IHH). At least 19 different mutations have been identified in this G-protein-coupled receptor, which consist mostly of missense mutations. The Gln106Arg and Arg262Gln mutations comprise nearly half of the identified alleles. Most mutations impair ligand binding and all compromise cell signaling events. Some of the mutations also adversely affect activation of gonadotropin subunit or *Gnrhr* gene promoters. Interestingly, a number of the mutant GnRHRs can be rescued in vitro from misfolding and degradation within the cell by the addition of a GnRHR antagonist IN3. Most affected patients have compound heterozygous *GNRHR* mutations that may cause either complete IHH (no evidence of puberty) or incomplete IHH (partial evidence of puberty), although some genotypes are associated with mild disease in some families and severe disease in others. *GNRHR* mutations also appear to cause constitutional delay of puberty, and one genotype (homozygosity for Gln106Arg) may be reversible in patients with IHH. Mutations in the human *GNRHR* gene have contributed greatly to the understanding of normosmic IHH, as well as the structure and function of the GnRHR.

It has been a decade since mutations in the human gonadotropin-releasing hormone receptor gene *(GNRHR)* were first identified. The discovery that the receptor *GNRHR*, rather than the ligand *GNRH1*, was the first gene found to cause autosomal recessive idiopathic hypogonadotropic hypogonadism (IHH) [1, 2] was somewhat surprising. This was particularly true given that the hypogonadal mouse, a naturally occurring mouse with an IHH phenotype, demonstrated a *Gnrh1* gene deletion [3]. In this mouse, gonadal function was restored by transplanting functional gonadotropin-releasing hormone (GnRH) neurons or by gene therapy using the wild-type *Gnrh1* cDNA [4]. Several rare human *GNRH1* mutations have now been described (see Bouligand et al., this volume, pp. 111–120).

In this review, we will discuss the structure and function of the human GnRHR and describe each of the different identified *GNRHR* mutations in humans, along with their functional analyses. Lastly, we will examine the genotype/phenotype correlations and the prevalence of *GNRHR* gene mutations in patients with IHH/Kallmann syndrome (KS).

Human *GNRHR* Structure and Function

The human *GNRHR* gene spans 18.7 kb of genomic sequence on chromosome 4q13.2 and consists of three exons [5–7]. The GnRHR protein is a G-protein-coupled receptor that is expressed on the cell surface of pituitary gonadotrophs [8]. The *GNRHR* gene is also expressed in many other tissues including the placenta, brain, ovary, testis, endometrium, myometrium, prostate, kidney, and liver [9]. The encoded 328-amino acid protein (NP 000397) contains the characteristic seven transmembrane domains (TMDs), along with an N-terminal extracellular domain (ECD), three extracellular (ECL) and three intracellular (ICL) loops, but notably lacks a large intracellular cytoplasmic tail (fig. 1). The ECDs and/or TMDs are involved in the formation of the ligand-binding pocket. Amino acid residues Asp^{98}, Asn^{102}, Lys^{121}, Asp^{302}, and Asn^{305} are thought to directly contact GnRH [10], whereas the cytoplasmic regions interact with G proteins and other intracellular regulatory proteins. Pulsatile GnRH released from hypophyseal-portal capillaries is delivered to the pituitary where it interacts with the *GNRHR* to initiate a cascade of events culminating in the synthesis and secretion of gonadotropins follicle-stimulating hormone (FSH) and luteinizing hormone (LH). Gonadotropins then stimulate the testes or ovaries to produce sex steroids and gametes.

Once the decapeptide GnRH binds to the GnRH receptor, cell signaling involves the G proteins, typically $G_{\alpha q}$, which activates phospholipase Cβ resulting in the production of second messengers inositol trisphosphate (IP_3), diacyl glycerol, and calcium with subsequent secretion of both FSH and LH [9]. However, additional G-proteins – $G_{\alpha s}$ (pituitary) and $G_{\alpha i}$ (cancer cells) – may be involved in GnRH signaling depending on the cell types [9]. $G_{\alpha s}$ stimulates and $G_{\alpha i}$ inhibits the adenylate cyclase/cyclic adenosine monophosphate (cAMP) pathway. There is also evidence that the pulse frequency of GnRH plays a large role in determining which of the two gonadotropins is released, with faster GnRH pulses preferentially stimulating LH release and slower pulses favoring FSH secretion [11]. Although a second *GNRHR* gene has been identified in many species, in the human ortholog on chromosome 1q21, the open reading frame is disrupted by a frameshift resulting in a truncated protein. However, it is interesting that this gene is transcriptionally active and may interfere with normal processing of the type I receptor in the nucleus, endoplasmic reticulum, or Golgi [12].

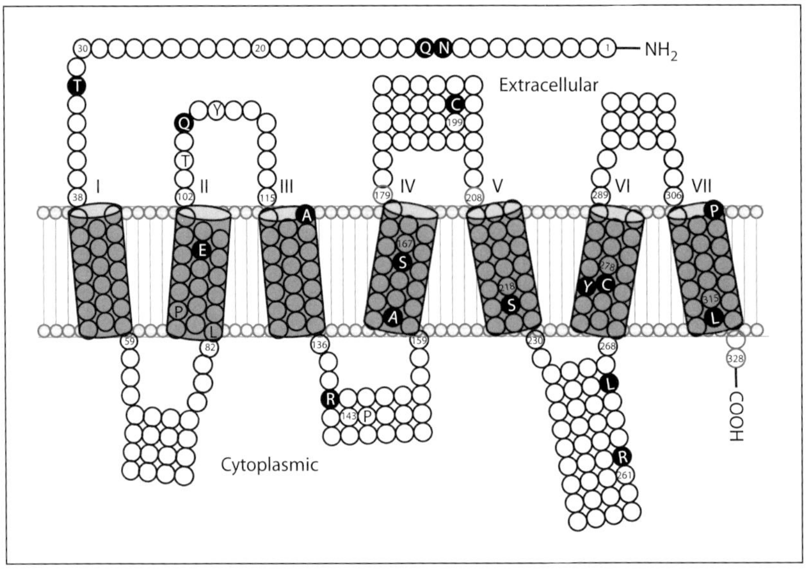

Fig. 1. Topology diagram of the amino acid sequence of the human GnRHR protein that was generated using the HMMTOP transmembrane topology prediction server [54, 55]. The predicted seven TMDs are indicated as cylinders, numbered I–VII. Also shown are the predicted ECLs above and the ICLs below the TMDs. All missense mutations confirmed by in vitro analysis and one non-sense mutation (L314X) are depicted in white amino acid abbreviations on black circles. Missense mutations not studied in vitro are depicted in black letters on white or shaded circles. Residue numbers are given at the boundary of TMDs and at other locations near mutated residues.

First Identification of *GNRHR* Mutations

Mutations in the *GNRHR* gene were identified by two independent groups utilizing different strategies [1, 2]. De Roux et al. [1] hypothesized that partial loss of function mutations would be expected in patients with incomplete pubertal development similar to those seen with LH receptor and thyroid stimulating hormone receptor mutations. They studied a 22-year-old male with delayed puberty at 18, who had decreased libido, small (8 ml) testes (normal testes size 15–25 ml), and a small penis. His testosterone was low at 80 ng/dl (normal 260–690 ng/dl) and his gonadotropins were low. LH pulse frequency was normal, but the amplitude was decreased. His semen analysis revealed a normal sperm concentration of 39 million/ml with low motility (5%). He was found to harbor compound heterozygous *GNRHR* mutations Gln106Arg/Arg262Gln (fig. 1), which were then studied in vitro upon transfection into COS-7 cells. The Gln106Arg mutation in ECL1 markedly impaired GnRH agonist binding to the receptor. Both the Gln106Arg and the Arg262Gln in ICL3 lowered IP_3 production by 50% and the IP_3 efficiency 50-fold in that 50 times the dose of GnRH agonist was needed to effect a 50% rise in IP_3 production [1]. This male had a sister, who had thelarche at age 14 years and menarche at age 18 (with only one period). Similar to her brother, she exhibited compound heterozygosity for these two mutations [9]. The unaffected parents were heterozygous for either of the two mutations and an unaffected daughter was heterozygous, indicating autosomal recessive inheritance.

Just over a month later, Layman et al. [2] reported a family with compound heterozygous *GNRHR* mutations. They reasoned that since *GNRH1* mutations had not yet been identified and that some IHH patients were resistant to GnRH treatment, the *GNRHR* gene represented a promising candidate gene for mutations in IHH. Forty-six normosmic IHH patients were studied using polymerase chain reaction (PCR) and denaturing gradient gel electrophoresis. Two variant fragments were identified in one family with 4 severely affected IHH patients [2]. Upon DNA sequencing, compound heterozygous *GNRHR* mutations Arg262Gln/Tyr284Cys (fig. 1) were identified in all 4 affected patients, but not in unaffected sibs (parents were deceased), indicating autosomal recessive inheritance.

The proband was a 30-year-old female without any breast development (Tanner 1). She had two sisters, ages 17 and 21, both with Tanner 1 breasts, and a brother who did not shave and had a serum testosterone of 75 ng/dl (he did not permit a genital exam). Neither mutation had any effect upon receptor binding; however, similar to De Roux et al. [1], the Arg262Gln impaired signal transduction following transfection using COS-1 cells. The Arg262Gln demonstrated a 25% reduction in receptor expression, a 40% reduction in IP_3 production, and a 10-fold increase in the amount of GnRH agonist needed to effect a 50% maximal increase in IP_3 production. The Tyr284Cys in TMD7 had an even more pronounced detrimental effect upon GnRH signaling with an 80% reduction in receptor expression, a 75% reduction in IP_3 production, and a 20-fold increase in the amount of GnRH agonist to result in a 50% maximal IP_3 response [2].

These two publications set the tone for those which followed, underscoring the phenotypic variation in mutations. In the first family, both affected members displayed a phenotype of incomplete IHH, whereby some evidence of sexual development and reproductive potential was present [1]. This family had the combination of a mutation in the ECL1 (Gln106Arg) that affected binding and signal transduction and a mutation in ICL3 that impaired signal transduction. However, in the second family, there was no evidence of any pubertal development in any of the 4 affected individuals, as they had complete IHH [2]. Both alleles impaired signal transduction that resulted in a more severe phenotype. Two of the three mutations identified, Gln106Arg and the Arg262Gln, have been determined to represent the most common alleles in all reported cases of human *GNRHR* mutations [13].

Additional *GNRHR* Mutations in Humans

Following these two initial reports [1, 2], our review of the literature has revealed a total of 19 different *GNRHR* alleles, all confirmed by functional analyses, that have

Table 1. All (n = 19) different human *GNRHR* mutant alleles reported to date, including mutation location in the gene and protein, the number of times the allele has been reported, and the effects upon binding and IP_3 signaling

No.	Reference	Exon	Allele(s)	n	Protein	Binding	IP_3 signaling	Other
Missense mutations								
1	[23]	1	Asn10Lys	1	ECD	↓	↓	
2	[33]	1	Asn10Lys +Gln11Lys	1	ECD	↓	↓	
3	[21, 29]	1	Thr32Ile	1	ECD	↓	↓	
4	[20, 25]	1	Glu90Lys	2	TMD2	↓	↓	
5	[1, 17, 21–24]	1	Gln106Arg	13	ECL1	↓	↓	
6	[14, 26]	1	Ala129Asp	2	TMD3	↓	↓	
7	[23, 31]	1	Arg139His	4	TMD3/ ICL2	absent	↓	↓ receptor No.
8	[34]	1	Arg139Cys	2	TMD3/ ICL2	normal	↓	
9	[16]	1	Ser168Arg	2	TMD4	↓	↓	
10	[32]	1	Ala171Thr	1	TMD4	absent	↓	
11	[21, 29]	2	Cys200Tyr	1	ECL2	↓	↓	
12	[15]	2	Gln106Arg/ Ser217Arg	1	ECL1/ TMD5	↓	↓	
13	[1, 2, 14, 17, 21, 26, 35]	3	Arg262Gln	8	ICL3	normal	↓	
14	[21, 29]	3	Leu266Arg	2	ICL3	↓	↓	
15	[21, 29]	3	Cys279Tyr	2	TMD6	↓	↓	
16	[2]	3	Tyr284Cys	1	TMD7	normal	↓	
17	[33]	3	Pro320Leu	1	TMD7	absent	↓	
Other mutations								
18	[27]	IVS1	IVS1–1G→A	2	Exon2 skip	ND	ND	
19	[18]	3	Leu314X	1	TMD7	↓	↓	

Table 1. Continued

No.	Reference	Exon	Allele(s)	n	Protein	Binding	IP_3 signaling	Other
Other reported alleles not studied in vitro								
20	[38]	1	Leu83Val	1		ND	ND	
21	[38]	1	Pro96Ser	1		ND	ND	
22	[37]	1	Thr104Ile	1		ND	ND	
23	[37]	1	Tyr108Cys	1		ND	ND	
24	[39]	1	Pro146Ser	2		ND	ND	

Missense mutations are ordered by codon number. Five additional alleles (No. 20–24) have also been reported, but not studied in vitro. Only newly identified alleles were included from Cerrato et al. [38] since it was not possible to determine which patients with known causative alleles had been reported previously. ND= Not done.

been described in IHH patients (table 1; fig. 1) [13–36]. Of these confirmed mutant alleles, 17 were missense mutations, one was a nonsense mutation, and one was a splice site mutation (table 1). In addition, 5 missense mutations were identified which have not been studied in vitro, and are therefore, considered presumptive mutations (table 1) [37–39]. Of the confirmed mutations, 10 were found in exon 1, 2 were identified in exon 2, and 6 were seen in exon 3. The splice mutant was identified at the splice donor site in intron 1, which resulted in exon skipping [27]. Although concentrated in two exons, the mutations seem to be spread throughout most of the different domains of the protein – the ECD, ECL 1 and 2, TMD2–7, and ICL 3. Nevertheless, two mutations appear to be particularly common, even among different ethnic groups: Gln106Arg represents 13 of 48 (27.1%) mutant alleles and Arg262Gln constitutes 8/46 (17.4%) mutant alleles (table 1) [13]. It is interesting that only one new causative mutation, Arg139Cys [34], has been identified in the *GNRHR* since the 2005 report by Bhagavath et al. [13].

All the reported *GNRHR* mutations were identified by PCR-based methods and DNA sequencing. However, these techniques do not detect heterozygous intragenic deletions. Deletions (and duplications) would be missed by PCR and DNA sequencing if a deletion occurred outside the boundary defined by the primers since the other (normal) allele would be amplified. A number of techniques have been reported to determine if heterozygous intragenic deletions occur, such as multiplex ligation-dependent amplification (MLPA) [40]. However, in a study of 100 IHH/KS using MLPA, no intragenic deletions were identified in the *GNRHR*, or any of the other autosomal genes studied *(GNRH1*, *GPR54*, *NELF*, or *FGFR1*), suggesting that deletions are not as common as in some other genetic disorders [40].

Functional Analysis of Human *GNRHR* Mutations

Most *GNRHR* mutations were studied in vitro utilizing transfection of the wild type and mutant separately into COS cells since they do not express the *GNRHR* [1, 2]. Ligand binding studies were performed upon membrane fractions by radioreceptor assays using labeled and unlabeled GnRH agonist [1, 2]. IP_3 radioreceptor studies were also performed on cytosolic components using labeled and unlabeled IP_3 to determine second messenger production and efficiency [1, 2].

More recently, additional studies have been performed on some *GNRHR* mutants to determine more clearly the mechanisms involved in their dysfunction. Cellular localization has been analyzed using immunofluorescence in GH3 cells transfected with the wild type or mutant receptor [29]. The effect of the mutant receptor has also been studied with regard to the ability to activate promoters of the gonadotropin genes in GH3 cells, including the *Cga* (chorionic gonadotropin-α), FSH-β *(Fshb)*, and LH-β *(Lhb)* promoters using the corresponding promoter sequence cloned upstream to luciferase (Luc) reporter sequence [29]. Cyclic AMP-dependent activity has been studied by cloning the cAMP response element (CRE) upstream to Luc, and the MAPK pathway has been studied by determining extracellular signal-regulated kinase (ERK) phosphorylation by Western blot analysis [30]. Finally, the effect of the mutant *GNRHR* upon *Gnrhr*/Luc promoter activity was studied to determine the effects of the mutants upon its own expression [29].

Fourteen of 19 (73.6%) of the reported *GNRHR* mutations interfere with ligand binding, while all interfere with affect IP_3 signal transduction (table 1). If binding is reduced, signal transduction would also be predicted to be impaired. One of the 17 missense mutations was found to markedly reduce cell surface expression, but not binding. For this Arg139Cys mutation, expression was increased by the administration of IN3 (a GnRHR antagonist), which has been reported to rescue degradation when mutant, misfolded GnRHRs have been misrouted to the endoplasmic reticulum rather than the cell surface. Once there was a sufficient increase in mutant receptors, ligand binding assays were found to be normal [34]. Even though 14 of the 19 mutations interfered with binding to GnRH agonist, it is interesting that none of them appear to be residues known to bind to GnRH [9].

In addition to the phospholipase C pathway via $G_{\alpha q}$, GnRH signaling may occur by the $G_{\alpha s}$ pathway via protein kinase A/cAMP pathway and ERK activation [9]. Although both the Gln106Arg and Arg262Gln mutations had similar detrimental effects upon stimulation of the *Fshb* (14- and 15-fold, respectively) and the *Lhb* (8.8- and 8.1-fold, respectively) promoters, Arg262Gln had a more significant effect upon *Cga* and *Cre* promoter activity, and phosphorylation of ERK (table 2) [30]. These findings indicate that both mutations may have differential effects upon these pathways, further providing a better mechanistic understanding of the pathogenesis of these mutations. In addition, both Leu266Arg and Cys279 were unable to stimulate gonadotropin subunit or *GNRHR* promoter activity in vitro (table 2), while

Table 2. Other in vitro analyses of the mutant *GNRHR*s reported in patients with normosmic IHH

No.	Allele	Protein	*Fshb* P	*Lhb* P	*Cga* P	*Gnrhr* P	*Cre* P	ERK Phos	IN3 rescue
1	Asn10Lys	ECD							yes [43]
2	Asn10Lys +Gln11Lys	ECD							
3 [29]	Thr32Ile	ECD	↓4	↓2.2	↓3	↓3.3	↓1.5	↓11.8	yes [42]
4	Glu90Lys	TMD2							yes [42]
5 [30]	Gln106Arg	ECL1	↓14	↓8.8	↓3.8	↓2.2	↓2.7	↓2.7	yes [43]
6	Ala129Asp	TMD3							partial [43]
7	Arg139His	TMD3/ICL2							partial [43]
8	Arg139Cys	TMD3/ICL2							
9	Ser168Arg	TMD4							no [43]
10	Ala171Thr	TMD4							
11 [29]	Cys200Tyr	ECL2	none	↓3.4	↓4.5	none	↓3.9	none	partial [42, 43]
12	Ser217Arg	ECL1/TMD5							no [43]
13 [30]	Arg262Gln	ICL3	↓15	↓ 8.1	↓10.6	↓3.7	↓6.7	↓5.1	yes [42]
14 [29]	Leu266Arg	ICL3	none	none	none	none	none	none	partial [42, 43]
15 [29]	Cys279Tyr	TMD6	none	none	none	none	none	none	partial [42, 43]
16	Tyr284Cys	TMD7							yes [43]
17	Pro320Leu	TMD7							

The fold reduction in sensitivity (i.e. the fold increase in the ED_{50}) to the promoters (*Fshb, Lhb, Cga, Cre*) is shown, as well as the effects of the mutant receptor upon ERK phosphorylation with GnRH agonist administration, and whether or not rescue occurred with the administration of the *GNRHR* antagonist IN3. Numbering of the mutations is the same as in table 1. Only those studied are shown. References are included in the mutation No. column.

Cys200Tyr and Thr32Ile were able to stimulate gonadotropin subunit and *GNRHR* promoter activity, demonstrating the complexity of these mutants upon different signaling pathways [29].

Interestingly, studies utilizing site-directed mutagenesis and in vitro analysis have shown that some *GNRHR* mutations appear to act as dominant negative mutations [41]. Since rescue of the Glu90Lys mutation was accomplished by either deleting Lys191 or adding a carboxy-terminal sequence [25], 13 of the human *GNRHR* mutations were studied further [42, 43]. Most (11 of 13) of the mutations shown in table 1 can be rescued using the GnRHR antagonist IN3, which the authors suggested corrects improper trafficking of the misfolded, mutant receptors from degradation and allows them to assume their normal localization in the cell membrane (table 2). These findings do suggest that perhaps several different mechanisms could be involved in the pathophysiology of *GNRHR* mutations. Of note, a *Gnrhr* mutant mouse (created by ENU mutagenesis) has a phenotype consistent with IHH, but the mutant was not able to be rescued by IN3 [44].

Since most human *GNRHR* mutations are missense, we used SIFT (sorting intolerant from tolerant) [45], which is used to compare all of the amino acid residues from different species to assign a probability of whether an amino acid change is likely to be tolerated or not (table 3). If the $p < 0.05$ for a particular amino acid substitution, then it is predicted to be not tolerated. It is interesting that SIFT analysis predicted that only 9/17 of the reported missense mutations would not be tolerated, and therefore would be predicted to impair protein function. This analysis was based on the comparisons of 14 available species for which the *GNRHR* has been cloned. If more distant species are excluded, 12/17 (70.6%) of the demonstrated functional *GNRHR* mutations would have been predicted to be detrimental. Only one missense mutation (Ala184Pro) was found in SNP database, and as expected, it was predicted to be tolerated. SIFT has been successfully used by a number of investigators to identify potential mutations to further study by functional assays [45–47], but its predictive value is somewhat limited in the human *GNRHR* gene.

Genotype/Phenotype Correlation in *GNRHR* Mutations

In our analysis of reported *GNRHR* mutations, we identified 17 different reported genotypes, some of which were reported in two or three different families (table 4). These genotypes were grouped based upon severity into complete IHH (no evidence of puberty), incomplete IHH (partial evidence of puberty), constitutional delay of puberty, or not reported. As shown in table 4, 9/17 (52.9%) different genotypes (seen in 11 families) resulted in a phenotype of complete IHH, and 5/17 (29.4%) from 8 different families had incomplete IHH. Two genotypes (Gln106Arg/Arg262Gln and Gln106Arg/Leu266Arg) identified in five unrelated families could cause either complete or incomplete IHH. It is interesting that the one family with compound heterozygous Gln106Arg/Arg262Gln mutations and complete IHH also had a heterozygous *FGFR1* mutation (table 4) [48].

Given the small number of affected individuals with these different genotypes, it is difficult to make precise genotype/phenotype correlations. However, some genotype/phenotype correlations become apparent when examining table 4. Perhaps the most transparent is the Gln106Arg genotype reflecting mild disease. Of the 11 families with complete IHH, only two (2/11) have a Gln106Arg allele, while five of the seven families with incomplete IHH have this allele. In the 3 unrelated probands who had

Table 3. SIFT analysis for the *GNRHR* missense mutations using the following 14 species: human, mouse, rat, cow, dog, boar, platypus, monkey, chimpanzee, chicken, rabbit, trout, sheep, and *Caenorhabditis elegans*

No.	Exon	Mutation		SIFT 1	SIFT 2 and 3	SIFT 4	SIFT 5
		nucleotide	amino acid				
1	1	Asn10Lys	N10K	I			
2	1	Gln11Lys	Q11K	T			
3	1	Thr32Ile	T32I	I			
4	1	Glu90Lys	E90K	T	T	I	I
5	1	Gln106Arg	Q106R	T			
6	1	Ala129Asp	A129D	I			
7	1	Arg139His	R139H	I			
8	1	Arg139Cys	R139C	I			
9	1	Ser168Arg	S168R	T			
10	1	Ala171Thr	A171T	I			
11	2	Cys200Tyr	C200Y	T	I	I	I
12	2	Ser217Arg	S217R	T	T	T	I
13	3	Arg262Gln	R262Q	I			
14	3	Leu266Arg	L266R	I			
15	3	Cys279Tyr	C279Y	T			
16	3	Tyr284Cys	Y284C	T			
17	3	Pro320Leu	P320L	I			
Mutations not studied in vitro							
18	1	Leu83Val	L83V	I			
19	1	Pro96Ser	P96S	I			
20	1	Thr104Ile	T104I	I			
21	1	Tyr108Cys	Y108C	T			
22	1	Pro146Ser	P146S	T	I	I	I

SIFT 1 includes all 14 orthologs; SIFT 2 is without *C. elegans*; SIFT 3 is without *C. elegans* and trout; SIFT 4 is without *C. elegans*, trout, and chicken; SIFT 5 is without *C. elegans*, trout, chicken, and platypus

homozygosity for the Gln106Arg allele, some degree of sexual development was present in all, suggesting that this is a mild allele.

Two unrelated probands demonstrating compound heterozygosity for the Ala129Asp/Arg262Gln had complete IHH, lacking any identifiable signs of steroid production. In the family described by Caron et al. [14], 2 affected males had micropenis and bilateral cryptorchidism, and the female completely lacked breast development. Layman et al. [26] identified this same genotype in another unrelated male with complete IHH, but this affected male had prepubertal-sized, bilaterally descended testes with some spermatogenesis response to gonadotropin stimulation. Both unrelated probands with homozygosity for Arg139His also presented with complete IHH

Table 4. Genotype/phenotype correlations for patients with *GNRHR* mutations that have been supported by functional analysis

No.	Reference	Genotype	Phenotype	n	Sex	Ethnicity
Severe phenotype–complete IHH						
1	[14, 26]	Ala129Asp/Arg262Gln	complete complete	2	M, F M	NA Caucasian
2	[23, 31]	Arg139His (HMZ)	complete complete	2	F M	Brazilian NA
3	[18]	Leu314X/Gln106Arg	complete	1	F	NA
4	[27]	IVS1, G-A, -1	complete	1	F	Indian
5	[2]	Arg262Gln/ Tyr284Cys	complete	1	M, F	Caucasian
6	[16]	Ser168Arg (HMZ)	complete	1	M	NA
7	[21]	Thr32Ile/Cys200Tyr	complete	1	M	NA
8	[32]	Ala171Thr/Gln106Arg	complete	1	M	Caucasian
9	[20, 25]	Glu90Lys (HMZ)	complete	1	M	Mexican Mestizo
Intermediate phenotype within families						
10	[1, 17, 21]	Gln106Arg/Arg262Gln	incomplete complete[1]	2	M, F F, F	NA NA
11	[21, 36]	Gln106Arg/Leu266Arg	incomplete complete incomplete	3	F F F	NA Caucasian NA
Milder phenotype–incomplete IHH						
12	[21, 22, 24]	Gln106Arg (HMZ)	incomplete[2] incomplete incomplete[3]	3	M F M	NA NA NA
13	[15]	Arg262Gln/Gln106+Ser217Arg	incomplete	1	M, F	NA
14	[23]	Asn10Lys/Gln106Arg	incomplete	1	M, F	Brazilian
15	[33]	Asn10Lys+Gln11Lys/ Pro320Leu	incomplete	1	F	Caucasian
16	[35]	Arg262Gln (HMZ)	incomplete or CDP	1	M, M	Asian Indian
Unknown severity						
17	[21]	Cys279Tyr (HMZ)	unknown	1	M	NA

Mutations are categorized on the basis of disease severity (complete IHH; complete or incomplete IHH; incomplete IHH); the number of times the specific genotype has been reported in unrelated families, the sex of the proband within the family, and ethnicity. NA = Not available; M = male; F = female.

[1] Patient also had a heterozygous FGFR1 mutation [48].

[2] Patient had a spontaneous pregnancy (and therefore reversal) [24].

[3] Patient had spontaneous reversal with normal levels of testosterone and gonadotropins [22, 49].

(table 1). The other genotypes have only been reported once, making genotype/phenotype comparisons difficult.

As is common in most genetic diseases, clinical heterogeneity in phenotype was observed within families with *GNRHR* mutations. Some affected patients within the same family may show some signs of pubertal development, while others exhibit a total lack of pubertal development (complete IHH) [13]. Although all 4 sibs with Arg262Gln/Tyr284Cys compound heterozygous mutations had a complete absence of pubertal development, the response to exogenous GnRH varied among them [26]. This occurred despite the demonstration that both mutations markedly impaired IP_3 signal transduction (20-fold decrease for Tyr284Cys and 10-fold decrease for Arg262Gln) [2]. When a second dose of GnRH was given to 2 of these patients, all FSH and LH levels were higher than the responses after the initial dose, suggesting that some priming and function of the receptor occurs with these mutant *GNRHR*s [26]. Interestingly, the affected male also had a ring chromosome 21, and there was also another sister with Down syndrome, whose pubertal status was not ascertained [2, 19]. This variation in phenotype in different families or even within the same family is likely influenced by other modifier genes, epigenetic events, and environmental factors.

Other investigators have reported successful priming of the GnRHR, and even ovulation and pregnancy with exogenous GnRH [17, 24] or spontaneously [24] has been reported in a small number of patients. Although term deliveries have been reported, the risk of spontaneous abortion is also high. One female with compound heterozygosity for Gln106Arg/Arg262Gln had 3 children with gonadotropin stimulation, but her sister had three spontaneous abortions [17]. Another patient with homozygosity for the Gln106Arg mutation had several miscarriages and no term deliveries [24]. Nevertheless, term pregnancies have been reported in patients with GNRHR mutations, suggesting that receptor function is not mandatory for human pregnancy.

Now that the most severe phenotypes have been examined, it is reasonable to consider patients with a less severe phenotype. Lin et al. [35] described a homozygous Arg262Gln *GNRHR* mutation in a patient with constitutional delay of puberty (CDP) and his brother, who could either have CDP or IHH (this could be determined when he reaches age 18). It is less clear if *GNRHR* mutations cause adult-onset IHH, but this does appear to be reasonable. At least one IHH patient with homozygosity for Arg106Gln *GNRHR* mutation has been reported to have a spontaneous reversal of his IHH when treatment was discontinued [49]. This phenomenon was also reported in another patient with Gln106Arg homozygosity, who had reversal with a spontaneous pregnancy [24]. These very interesting findings suggest that perhaps IHH patients, particularly with mild mutations, could have their steroid treatment discontinued periodically to determine if pulsatile gonadotropin responses ensue without treatment.

Table 5. Studies of prevalence of *GNRHR* mutations

Reference	Sample size of IHH/KS	Mutations	Prevalence in nIHH	Method of analysis
[13]	185	3	3/85 (3.5%)	DGGE/ sequencing
[21]	108	5	5/48 (10.4%)	TGGE/sequencing
[56]	45	0	0/45 (0%)	SSCP/sequencing
[39]	26	0	0/26 0 (0%)	DNA sequencing
[57]	17	0	0/5(0%)	DNA sequencing
[34]	22	1	1/22 (4.5%)	DNA sequencing
Total	403	9/403 (1.5%)	9/231 (3.9%)	
Determination of heterozygous deletions				
[40]	100	no deletions	0	MLPA

To date, there have been no reported *GNRHR* mutations in 125 anosmic/hyposmic patients [13, 21]. DGGE = Denaturing gradient gel electrophoresis; TGGE = temperature gradient gel electrophoresis; SSCP = single-strand conformation polymorphism; nIHH = normosmic IHH.

Prevalence of Human *GNRHR* Mutations

GNRHR mutations cause autosomal recessive, normosmic IHH. Compound heterozygous *GNRHR* mutations were first found in a single proband (and affected siblings) from a total of 46 normosmic IHH patients for a prevalence of 2.2%. When only females were considered, then 1/14 (7.1%) were affected [2]. When this study was updated to include a sample of 185 IHH/KS patients by Bhagavath et al. [13], similar findings were seen. Findings from this largest study to date indicate that *GNRHR* mutations were found in 6–11% of IHH families, demonstrating clear autosomal recessive inheritance [13]. Another potential indicator of an autosomal recessive disease would be to determine the prevalence of *GNRHR* mutations in all unrelated females studied. Of the 34 female IHH patients, 2 (5.9%) were affected, making the prevalence slightly higher in female patients [13]. If only normosmic females were considered, 2/18 (11.1%) had *GNRHR* mutations. No *GNRHR* mutations were found in any of the presumed autosomal dominant or X-linked recessive families. In another study by Beranova et al. [21], 5/108 (4.6%) IHH patients had *GNRHR* mutations, including 5/48 (10.4%) with normosmic IHH, and none of 60 anosmic IHH (KS) patients [21].

In table 5, findings from available studies suggest that the prevalence of *GNRHR* mutations in all IHH/KS patients ranges between 2 and 5%. If all patients (normosmic, anosmic/hyposmic, and unknown) are included, 1.5% of patients had *GNRHR* mutations. To date, there have been no reports of *GNRHR* mutations in anosmic or hyposmic IHH patients (n = 125) [13, 21], indicating that GNRHR mutations are extremely rare in patients with disorders of olfaction. Overall, the prevalence of

GNRHR mutations in normosmic IHH patients is 3.9%, ranging from 0 to 10.4% (table 5). Although *GNRHR* mutations are inherited in an autosomal recessive fashion, this was not apparent from their pedigrees since no additional family members were affected. Since untreated IHH affects fertility, families typically do not contain a large number of affected individuals.

Although *GNRHR* mutations were initially thought to be the most common cause of normosmic IHH [1, 2, 13], it appears that the mutation frequency of two autosomal dominantly inherited genes FGFR1 (10%) [50, 51] and CHD7 (6%) appear more common and, interestingly, cause similar frequencies of both normosmic IHH and KS [46]. Autosomal recessive gene mutations have been reported in at least seven genes – *GNRHR*, *LEP*, *LEPR*, *PCSK1*, *GPR54*, and *PROKR2*, and *PROK2*, but only *GNRHR* mutations appear to be very common. Mutations in these other six genes have only been described in a few affected individuals [52, 53]. Mutations in the *GNRHR* gene constituted the first known autosomal recessive molecular cause of IHH [1, 2] and still play an important role in normosmic IHH. *TAC3* and *TACR3* mutations have also recently been reported to cause autosomal recessive IHH (see Semple and Topaloglu, this volume, pp. 133–141).

Acknowledgements

This study was supported by NIH grants HD33004 and HD040287 (L.C.L). We appreciate the help of Steven Walker, graduate student at MCG, for his preparation of figure 1.

References

1 de Roux N, Young J, Misrahi M, Genet R, Chanson P, Schaison G, Milgrom E: A family with hypogonadotropic hypogonadism and mutations in the gonadotropin-releasing hormone receptor. N Engl J Med 1997;337:1597–1602.

2 Layman LC, Cohen DP, Jin M, Xie J, Li Z, Reindollar RH, Bolbolan S, Bick DP, Sherins RJ, Duck LW, Musgrove LC, Sellers JC, Neill JD: Mutations in the gonadotropin-releasing hormone receptor gene cause hypogonadotropic hypogonadism. Nat Genet 1998;18:14–15.

3 Mason AJ, Hayflick JS, Zoeller T, Young WS, Phillips HS, Nikolics K, Seeburg PH: A deletion truncating the gonadotropin-releasing hormone gene is responsible for hypogonadism in the hpg mouse. Science 1986;234:1366–1371.

4 Mason AJ, Pitts SL, Nikolics K, Szonyi E, Wilcox JN, Seeburg PH, Stewart TA: The hypogonadal mouse: reproductive functions restored by gene therapy. Science 1986;234:1372–1378.

5 Kakar SS, Musgrove LC, Devor DC, Sellers JC, Neill JD: Cloning, sequencing, and expression of human gonadotropin releasing hormone (GnRH) receptor. Biophys Biochem Res Commun 1992;189:289–295.

6 Fan NC, Jeung E-B, Peng C, Olofsson JI, Krisinger J, Leung PCK: The human gonadotropin-releasing hormone (GnRH) receptor gene: cloning, genomic organization and chromosomal assignment. Mol Cell Endocrinol 1994;103:R1–R6.

7 Kaiser UB, Dushkin H, Altherr MR, Beier DR, Chin WW: Chromosomal location of the gonadotropin-releasing hormone receptor gene to human chromosome 4q13.1-q21.1 and mouse chromosome 5. Genomics 1994;20:506–508.

8 Fan NC, Peng C, Krisinger J, Leung PC: The human gonadotropin-releasing hormone receptor gene: complete structure including multiple promoters, transcription initiation sites, and polyadenylation signals. Mol Cell Endocrinol 1995;107:R1–R8.

9 Bédécarrats GY, Kaiser UB: Mutations in the human gonadotropin-releasing hormone receptor: insights into receptor biology and function. Semin Reprod Med 2007;25:368–378.
10 Millar RP, Lu ZL, Pawson AJ, Flanagan CA, Morgan K, Maudsley SR: Gonadotropin-releasing hormone receptors. Endocr Rev 2004;25:235–275.
11 Kaiser UB, Jakubowiak A, Steinberger A, Chin WW: Differential effects of gonadotropin-releasing hormone (GnRH) pulse frequency on gonadotropin subunit and GnRH receptor messenger ribonucleic acid levels in vitro. Endocrinology 1997;138:1224–1231.
12 Pawson AJ, Maudsley S, Morgan K, Davidson L, Naor Z, Millar RP: Inhibition of human type i gonadotropin-releasing hormone receptor (GnRHR) function by expression of a human type II GnRHR gene fragment. Endocrinology 2005;146:2639–2649.
13 Bhagavath B, Ozata M, Ozdemir IC, Bolu E, Bick DP, Sherins RJ, Layman LC: The prevalence of gonadotropin-releasing hormone receptor mutations in a large cohort of patients with hypogonadotropic hypogonadism. Fertil Steril 2005;84:951–957.
14 Caron P, Chauvin S, Christin-Maitre S, Bennet A, Lahlou N, Counis R, Bouchard P, Kottler M-L: Resistance of hypogonadotropic patients with mutated GnRH receptor genes to pulsatile GnRH administration. J Clin Endocrinol Metab 1999;84:990–996.
15 de Roux N, Young J, Brailly-Tabard S, Misrahi M, Milgrom E, Chaison G: The same molecular defects of the gonadotropin-releasing hormone determine a variable degree of hypogonadism in affected kindred. J Clin Endocrinol Metab 1999;84:567–572.
16 Pralong FP, Gomez F, Castillo E, Cotecchia S, Abuin L, Aubert ML, Portmann L, Gaillard RC: Complete hypogonadotropic hypogonadism associated with a novel inactivating mutation of the gonadotropin-releasing hormone receptor. J Clin Endocrinol Metab 1999;84:3811–3816.
17 Seminara SB, Beranova M, Oliveira LM, Martin KA, Crowley WF Jr, Hall JE: Successful use of pulsatile gonadotropin-releasing hormone (GnRH) for ovulation induction and pregnancy in a patient with GnRH receptor mutations. J Clin Endocrinol Metab 2000;85:556–562.
18 Kottler ML, Chauvin S, Lahlou N, Harris CE, Johnston CJ, Lagarde JP, Bouchard P, Farid NR, Counis R: A new compound heterozygous mutation of the gonadotropin-releasing hormone receptor (L314X, Q106R) in a woman with complete hypogonadotropic hypogonadism: chronic estrogen administration amplifies the gonadotropin defect. J Clin Endocrinol Metab 2000;85:3002–3008.
19 Layman LC, McDonough PG, Cohen DP, Maddox M, Tho SP, Reindollar R: Familial gonadotropin-releasing hormone resistance and hypogonadotropic hypogonadism in a family with multiple affected individuals. Fertil Steril 2001;75:1148–1155.
20 Söderlund D, Canto P, de la Chesnaye E, Ulloa-Aguirre A, Méndez JP: A novel homozygous mutation in the second transmembrane domain of the gonadotrophin-releasing hormone receptor gene. Clin Endocrinol (Oxf) 2001;54:493–498.
21 Beranova M, Oliveira LM, Bédécarrats GY, Schipani E, Vallejo M, Ammini AC, Quintos JB, Hall JE, Martin KA, Hayes FJ, Pitteloud N, Kaiser UB, Crowley WF Jr, Seminara SB: Prevalence, phenotypic spectrum, and modes of inheritance of gonadotropin-releasing hormone receptor mutations in idiopathic hypogonadotropic hypogonadism. J Clin Endocrinol Metab 2001;86:1580–1588.
22 Pitteloud N, Boepple PA, DeCruz S, Valkenburgh SB, Crowley WF Jr, Hayes FJ: The fertile eunuch variant of idiopathic hypogonadotropic hypogonadism: spontaneous reversal associated with a homozygous mutation in the gonadotropin-releasing hormone receptor. J Clin Endocrinol Metab 2001;86:2470–2475.
23 Costa EM, Bédécarrats GY, Mendonca BB, Arnhold IJ, Kaiser UB, Latronico AC: Two novel mutations in the gonadotropin-releasing hormone receptor gene in Brazilian patients with hypogonadotropic hypogonadism and normal olfaction. J Clin Endocrinol Metab 2001;86:2680–2686.
24 Dewailly D, Boucher A, Decanter C, Lagarde JP, Counis R, Kottler ML: Spontaneous pregnancy in a patient who was homozygous for the Q106R mutation in the gonadotropin-releasing hormone receptor gene. Fertil Steril 2002;77:1288–1291.
25 Maya-Nunez G, Janovick JA, Ulloa-Aguirre A, Soderlund D, Conn PM, Mendez JP: Molecular basis of hypogonadotropic hypogonadism: restoration of mutant (E(90)K) GnRH receptor function by a deletion at a distant site. J Clin Endocrinol Metab 2002;87:2144–2149.
26 Layman LC, Cohen DP, Xie J, Smith GD: Clinical phenotype and infertility treatment in a male with hypogonadotropic hypogonadism due to mutations Ala129Asp/Arg262Gln of the gonadotropin-releasing hormone receptor. Fertil Steril 2002;78:1317–1320.
27 Silveira LF, Stewart PM, Thomas M, Clark DA, Bouloux PM, MacColl GS: Novel homozygous splice acceptor site GnRH receptor (GnRHR) mutation: human GnRHR 'knockout'". J Clin Endocrinol Metab 2002;87:2973–2977.
28 Bédécarrats GY, Kaiser UB: Differential regulation of gonadotropin subunit gene promoter activity by pulsatile gonadotropin-releasing hormone (GnRH) in perifused L beta T2 cells: role of GnRH receptor concentration. Endocrinology 2003;144:1802–1811.

29 Bédécarrats GY, Linher KD, Janovick JA, Beranova M, Kada F, Seminara SB, Michael Conn P, Kaiser UB: Four naturally occurring mutations in the human GnRH receptor affect ligand binding and receptor function. Mol Cell Endocrinol 2003;205:51–64.

30 Bédécarrats GY, Linher KD, Kaiser UB: Two common naturally occurring mutations in the human gonadotropin-releasing hormone (GnRH) receptor have differential effects on gonadotropin gene expression and on GnRH-mediated signal transduction. J Clin Endocrinol Metab 2003;88:834–843.

31 Wolczynski S, Laudanski P, Jarzabek K, Mittre H, Lagarde JP, Kottler ML: A case of complete hypogonadotropic hypogonadism with a mutation in the gonadotropin-releasing hormone receptor gene. Fertil Steril 2003;79:442–444.

32 Karges B, Karges W, Mine M, Ludwig L, Kuhne R, Milgrom E, de Roux N: Mutation Ala(171)Thr stabilizes the gonadotropin-releasing hormone receptor in its inactive conformation, causing familial hypogonadotropic hypogonadism. J Clin Endocrinol Metab 2003;88:1873–1879.

33 Meysing AU, Kanasaki H, Bédécarrats GY, Acierno JS Jr, Conn PM, Martin KA, Seminara SB, Hall JE, Crowley WF Jr, Kaiser UB: GNRHR mutations in a woman with idiopathic hypogonadotropic hypogonadism highlight the differential sensitivity of luteinizing hormone and follicle-stimulating hormone to gonadotropin-releasing hormone. J Clin Endocrinol Metab 2004;89:3189–3198.

34 Topaloglu AK, Lu ZL, Farooqi IS, Mungan NO, Yuksel B, O'Rahilly S, Millar RP: Molecular genetic analysis of normosmic hypogonadotropic hypogonadism in a Turkish population: identification and detailed functional characterization of a novel mutation in the gonadotropin-releasing hormone receptor gene. Neuroendocrinology 2006;84:301–308.

35 Lin L, Conway GS, Hill NR, Dattani MT, Hindmarsh PC, Achermann JC: A homozygous R262Q mutation in the gonadotropin-releasing hormone receptor presenting as constitutional delay of growth and puberty with subsequent borderline oligospermia. J Clin Endocrinol Metab 2006;91:5117–5121.

36 Quintos JB, Krotz S, Vogiatzi MG, Kralickova M, New MI: Partial hypogonadotropic hypogonadism associated with the Leu266Arg and GlN 106Arg mutations of the gonadotropin-releasing hormone receptor. J Pediatr Endocrinol Metab 2009;22:181–185.

37 Antelli A, Baldazzi L, Balsamo A, Pirazzoli P, Nicoletti A, Gennari M, Cicognani A: Two novel GnRHR gene mutations in two siblings with hypogonadotropic hypogonadism. Eur J Endocrinol 2006; 155:201–205.

38 Cerrato F, Shagoury J, Kralickova M, Dwyer A, Falardeau J, Ozata M, Van Vliet G, Bouloux P, Hall JE, Hayes FJ, Pitteloud N, Martin KA, Welt C, Seminara SB: Coding sequence analysis of GNRHR and GPR54 in patients with congenital and adult-onset forms of hypogonadotropic hypogonadism. Eur J Endocrinol 2006;155(suppl 1):S3–S10.

39 Vagenakis GA, Sgourou A, Papachatzopoulou A, Kourounis G, Papavassiliou AG, Georgopoulos NA: The gonadotropin-releasing hormone (GnRH)-1 gene, the GnRH receptor gene, and their promoters in patients with idiopathic hypogonadotropic hypogonadism with or without resistance to GnRH action. Fertil Steril 2005;84:1762–1765.

40 Pedersen-White JR, Chorich LP, Bick DP, Sherins RJ, Layman LC: The prevalence of intragenic deletions in patients with idiopathic hypogonadotropic hypogonadism and Kallmann syndrome. Mol Hum Reprod 2008;14:367–370.

41 Brothers SP, Cornea A, Janovick JA, Conn PM: Human loss-of-function gonadotropin-releasing hormone receptor mutants retain wild-type receptors in the endoplasmic reticulum: molecular basis of the dominant-negative effect. Mol Endocrinol 2004;18:1787–1797.

42 Janovick JA, Maya-Nunez G, Conn PM: Rescue of hypogonadotropic hypogonadism-causing and manufactured GnRH receptor mutants by a specific protein-folding template: misrouted proteins as a novel disease etiology and therapeutic target. J Clin Endocrinol Metab 2002;87:3255–3262.

43 Leanos-Miranda A, Janovick JA, Conn PM: Receptor-misrouting: an unexpectedly prevalent and rescuable etiology in gonadotropin-releasing hormone receptor-mediated hypogonadotropic hypogonadism. J Clin Endocrinol Metab 2002;87:4825–4828.

44 Pask AJ, Kanasaki H, Kaiser UB, Conn PM, Janovick JA, Stockton DW, Hess DL, Justice MJ, Behringer RR: A novel mouse model of hypogonadotrophic hypogonadism: N-ethyl-N-nitrosourea-induced gonadotropin-releasing hormone receptor gene mutation. Mol Endocrinol 2005;19:972–81.

45 Ng PC, Henikoff S: SIFT: predicting amino acid changes that affect protein function. Nucleic Acids Res 2003;31:3812–3814.

46 Kim HG, Kurth I, Lan F, Meliciani I, Wenzel W, Eom SH, Kang GB, Rosenberger G, Tekin M, Ozata M, Bick DP, Sherins RJ, Walker SL, Shi Y, Gusella JF, Layman LC: Mutations in CHD7, encoding a chromatin-remodeling protein, cause idiopathic hypogonadotropic hypogonadism and Kallmann syndrome. Am J Hum Genet 2008;83:511–519.

47 Raevaara TE, Korhonen MK, Lohi H, et al: Functional significance and clinical phenotype of non-truncating mismatch repair variants of MLH1. Gastroenterology 2005;129:537–549.

48 Pitteloud N, Quinton R, Pearce SH, et al: Digenic mutations account for variable phenotypes in idiopathic hypogonadotropic hypogonadism. J Clin Invest 2007;117:457–463.
49 Raivio T, Falardeau J, Dwyer AA, Quinton R, Hayes FJ, Hughes VA, Cole LW, Pearce SH, Lee H, Boepple P, Crowley WF Jr, Pitteloud N: Reversal of idiopathic hypogonadotropic hypogonadism. N Engl J Med 2007;357:863–873.
50 Pitteloud N, Acierno JS Jr, Meysing A, Eliseenkova AV, Ma J, Ibrahimi OA, Metzger DL, Hayes FJ, Dwyer AA, Hughes VA, Yialamas M, Hall JE, Grant E, Mohammadi M, Crowley WF Jr: Mutations in fibroblast growth factor receptor 1 cause both Kallmann syndrome and normosmic idiopathic hypogonadotropic hypogonadism. Proc Natl Acad Sci USA 2006;103:6281–6286.
51 Pitteloud N, Meysing A, Quinton R, Acierno JS Jr, Dwyer AA, Plummer L, Fliers E, Boepple P, Hayes FJ, Seminara SB, Hughes VA, Ma J, Bouloux PM, Mohammadi M, Crowley WF Jr: Mutations in fibroblast growth factor receptor 1 cause Kallmann syndrome with a wide spectrum of reproductive phenotypes. Mol Cell Endocrinol 2006;254–255:60–69.
52 Layman LC: Human gene mutations causing infertility. J Med Genet 2002;39:153–161.
53 Beier DR, Dluhy RG: Bench and bedside – the G protein-coupled receptor GPR54 and puberty. N Engl J Med 2003;349:1589–1592.
54 Tusnady GE, Simon I: Principles governing amino acid composition of integral membrane proteins: application to topology prediction. J Mol Biol 1998; 283:489–506.
55 Tusnady GE, Simon I: The HMMTOP transmembrane topology prediction server. Bioinformatics 2001;17:849–850.
56 Lanfranco F, Gromoll J, von Eckardstein S, Herding EM, Nieschlag E, Simoni M: Role of sequence variations of the GnRH receptor and G protein-coupled receptor 54 gene in male idiopathic hypogonadotropic hypogonadism. Eur J Endocrinol 2005;153:845–852.
57 Trarbach EB, Baptista MT, Garmes HM, Hackel C: Molecular analysis of KAL-1, GnRH-R, NELF and EBF2 genes in a series of Kallmann syndrome and normosmic hypogonadotropic hypogonadism patients. J Endocrinol 2005;187:361–368.

Lawrence C. Layman, MD
Section of Reproductive Endocrinology, Infertility, and Genetics
Department of Obstetrics and Gynecology, Medical College of Georgia
1120 15th Street, Augusta, GA 30912–3360 (USA)
Tel. +1 706 7213832, Fax +1 706 7216830, E-Mail llayman@mcg.edu

Quinton R (ed): Kallmann Syndrome and Hypogonadotropic Hypogonadism.
Front Horm Res. Basel, Karger, 2010, vol 39, pp 111–120

Hypogonadotropic Hypogonadism and *GNRH1* Mutations in Mice and Humans

Jérôme Bouligand[a,b] · Cristina Ghervan[d] · Anne Guiochon-Mantel[a,b] · Jacques Young[a,c]

[a]Université Paris-Sud 11 et INSERM U693, Faculté de Médecine Paris Sud, [b]Service de Génétique Moléculaire, Pharmacogénétique et Hormonologie, and [c]Service d'Endocrinologie et des Maladies de la Reproduction, Centre Hospitalier Universitaire de Bicêtre, Assistance Publique Hôpitaux de Paris, Paris, France; [d]Endocrinology Department, University of Medicine and Pharmacy Iuliu Hatieganu, Cluj-Napoca, Romania

Abstract

The neuropeptide gonadotropin-releasing hormone (GnRH) plays a key regulatory role in mammalian reproduction. It is synthesized by hypothalamic neurons and released from nerve endings into the portal circulation. After binding to membrane GnRH type 1 receptors on gonadotropic cells of the anterior pituitary, it stimulates the synthesis and release of luteinizing hormone and follicle-stimulating hormone. These two peptides travel through the general circulation to the gonads, where they stimulate the synthesis and secretion of sex steroid hormones and trigger gametogenesis. The discovery in 1977 of a hypogonadal mouse lacking GnRH (hpg mice) and, in 1986, that the *gnrh1* gene was deleted in this mouse, suggested that *GNRH1* mutations might also cause human congenital idiopathic (or isolated) hypogonadotropic hypogonadism. This was finally demonstrated in 2009.

Historical Perspective

The idea that hormones produced by the central nervous system could regulate reproduction was first raised by Crowe et al. [1] early in the 20th century. These researchers elegantly demonstrated that disruption of the hypothalamic-pituitary connection could prevent onset of puberty in dogs. The initial explanation for this observation was the possible existence of direct 'neurohumoral' input from the central neural system to the anterior pituitary. A few decades later, Geoffrey W. Harris effectively demonstrated neurohumoral hypothalamic control of anterior pituitary hormone secretion. Harris observed an unusual capillary system (a portal system of blood vessels) connecting the ventral hypothalamus to the anterior pituitary lobe [2] and speculated that it could serve to convey hypothalamic factors that trigger the release of anterior pituitary hormones [3]. He confirmed the importance of this vascular link in experiments using a variety of surgical and electrophysiological techniques; in particular, he showed that pituitary stalk section interrupted estrous cycling in the rat [3]. In a paradigm of simplicity, he and others found that transplanting pituitary tissue into the sella turcica, directly below the median eminence, in hypophysectomized female rats resulted in revascularization by portal vessels and fully restored pituitary function; in contrast, this did not occur if the pituitary was transplanted at a distance from this site and revascularized by systemic vessels [2–4]. Finally, after detecting luteinizing-hormone-releasing factor (LRF) in the median eminence with an elegant bioassay, in which he triggered an ovulatory response in rabbits by intrapituitary infusion of median eminence extracts, Harris began to purify LRF from the same tissue [2–4].

The existence of hypothalamic peptide messengers was fully validated in 1971 by the purification, isolation and structural characterization of gonadotropin-releasing hormone (GnRH; LRF) by the teams of Schally and Guillemin [5, 6], only 2 years after the tripeptide structure of TRH, another hypophysiotropic hypothalamic hormone, had been discovered. A few years after these discoveries, in a series of physiological studies involving non-human primates, Knobil [7] demonstrated the pulsatile nature of endogenous hypothalamic GnRH release [7], each GnRH pulse being associated with electrical activity in the arcuate nucleus of the hypothalamus, and being followed almost immediately by a pulse of luteinizing hormone (LH) secretion, as measured in the jugular vein. Then, using a rhesus monkey model with hypothalamic lesions that abolished gonadotropin release by the pituitary gland, Knobil's team showed that intermittent administration of exogenous GnRH, once per hour (the physiological frequency of gonadotropin release in these monkeys) re-established pituitary gonadotropin secretion, whereas constant infusion of GnRH failed to do so [8].

Cloning and Characterization of the Human *GNRH1* Gene

In 1984, Seeburg and Adelman [9] isolated and cloned both genomic and complementary DNA encoding the precursor of human GnRH. The complete gene nucleotide sequence was determined by the same group [10], who showed that the gene coded for a 92-amino-acid pre-prohormone encompassing both the decapeptide GnRH and GnRH-associated peptide (GAP), composed of 56 amino acids [11] (fig. 1). On the basis of in vitro and in vivo experiments, the same group claimed at the time that GAP corresponded to PIF (prolactin-release inhibiting factor; see below) [12].

The human gene encoding GnRH and GAP was designated '*GNRH1*' by the HUGO gene nomenclature committee (HGNC: 4419). *GNRH1* was located, by FISH and Southern blot, on the short arm of chromosome 8 at the 8p21-p11.2 locus [13], and was shown to span almost 6 kb, following the orientation of the negative strand of chromosome 8.

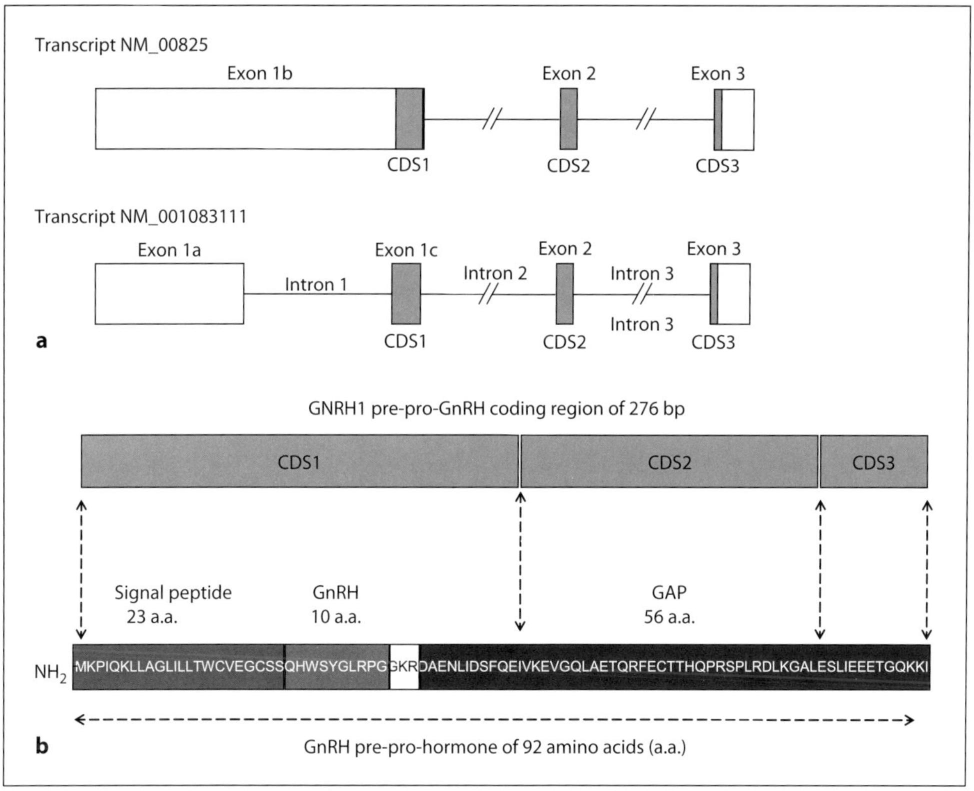

Fig. 1. *GNRH1* transcripts and pre-pro-GnRH. **a** The two main *GNRH1* transcription variants are due to alternative splicing of the first intron. Variant NM_00825 has only three exons, owing to retention of the first intron, and is expressed mainly in the placenta. Variant NM_001083111, with four exons, is the most abundant form in the hypothalamus. Exons are represented by quadrangles and coding regions (CDS) are shaded. Introns are represented by lines. **b** *GNRH1* coding regions (CDS 1–3, see **a**) aligned with pre-pro-GnRH.

Several *GNRH1* transcripts have since been described. First, it was shown that alternative splicing occurred, with the placental transcript comprising three exons and the hypothalamic one comprising all four exons (fig. 1a) [10]. *GNRH1* was then found to possess both upstream and downstream transcription start sites [14]. The former lacked the usual TATA and CAAT elements present in RNA polymerase II promoters, contrary to the usual downstream transcription start site. The upstream transcription start site was found to play a significant role in reproductive tissues such as placenta, mammary gland, testis and ovary [14], as well as breast cancer cell lines [15], whereas the downstream transcription start site is more crucial to GnRH expression in the hypothalamus (see below) [14]. Splicing, and the nature of the transcription start site, were found to be influenced by regulatory elements expressed in different cellular contexts, thus explaining the different relative expression of the various transcripts in the hypothalamus and in non-neuronal tissues [11, 16]. The two main GNRH1 transcript variants, validated by the National Center for Biotechnological Information, are shown in figure 1a. These two variants (NM_00825 and NM_001083111) arise through alternative splicing, with retention of the first intron preceding the coding region. Transcript NM_00825, in which intron 1 is not spliced, is preferentially detected in extra-hypothalamic tissue such as placenta, while transcript NM_001083111 is most abundant in the hypothalamus [10]. The exact function of GnRH expressed in extra-hypothalamic tissues is unknown, as are the hypothalamic or placental factors that direct differential splicing of the GnRH gene [17, 18]. These transcripts are probably translated into the same protein, as variations in splicing and in the transcription initiation sites only concern noncoding regions of the gene. The coding nucleotide sequences of GNRH1 and the 92-amino-acid pre-prohormone are aligned in figure 1b.

Hpg Mice, a Natural Model of Congenital Hypothalamic Hypogonadotropic Hypogonadism

In 1977, Cattanach et al. [19] published a seminal *Nature* paper describing a natural mutant mouse, where adults of both sexes exhibited complete hypogonadism. They demonstrated that this phenotype was related to hypothalamic GnRH deficiency and to the resulting reduction in pituitary LH and follicle-stimulating hormone content and in circulating gonadotropin levels [19] (fig. 2). Earlier evidence of a causal relationship between hypogonadotropic hypogonadism and GnRH deficiency in hpg mice was provided by both Krieger and Gibson and their colleagues [20, 21] who showed that grafts of normal fetal brain tissue from the preoptic region (which contains the majority of GnRH neurons in rodents), when placed in the third ventricle, reversed the endocrine deficiencies of both male and female hpg mice [20, 21].

In 1986, Mason et al. [22] demonstrated that the hereditary autosomal recessive hypogonadotropic hypogonadism in hpg mice was caused by a deletion of 33.5 kb encompassing the distal half of *gnrh1*. The partially deleted gene lacking the two exons that encode most of the GAP peptide (fig. 1) was transcriptionally active, as shown by in situ hybridization of hpg hypothalamic tissue sections, but translationally inactive since the peptide was undetectable by immunocytochemistry and radioimmunoassay with antibodies against different sections of the GnRH precursor [22]. The same group, using transgenic techniques, showed that restoring the normal *Gnrh1* gene in hpg mice led to full recovery of pituitary and gonadal functions [23], proving the crucial role of *Gnrh1* in hypothalamic control of rodent reproduction.

As indicated above, analysis of the hpg mouse *gnrh1* gene revealed a large deletion resulting in a truncated gene possessing only the promoter region, the first two exons encoding the signal peptide, the GnRH decapeptide itself, and the first 11 amino acid residues of GAP (fig. 1). But this mutation left the region encoding the GnRH decapeptide intact, leaving the mechanism underlying the hypogonadism of hpg mice unresolved. One possibility was that this gene truncation generated a nonfunctional

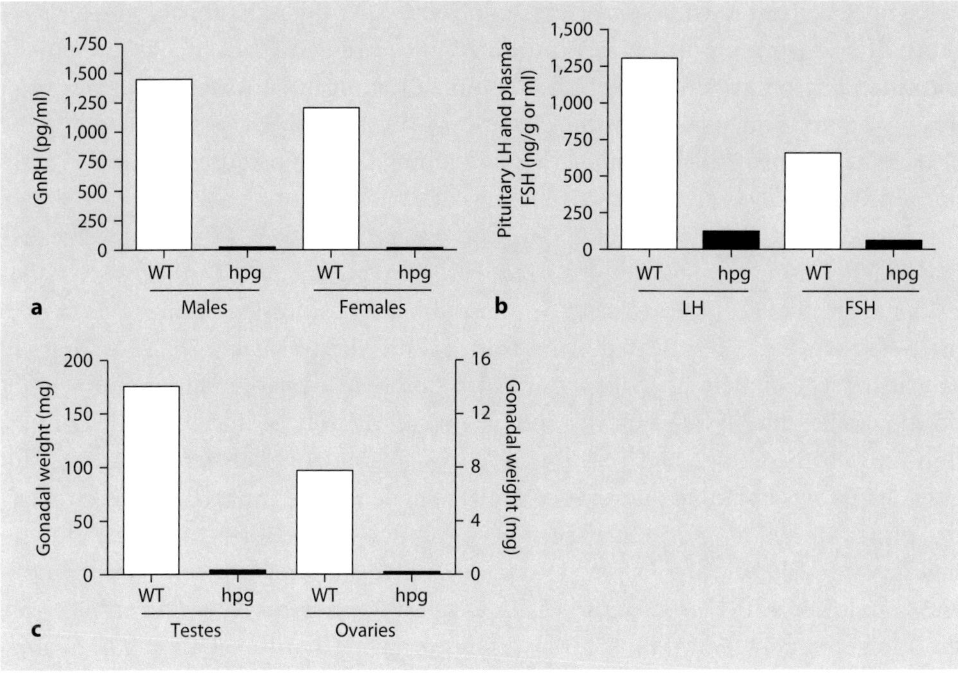

Fig. 2. GnRH deficiency and hypogonadotropic hypogonadism in the hpg mouse, as described by Cattanach et al. [19]. Comparison between wild-type (WT) and hpg mice. **a** GnRH content in the hypothalamus. **b** Pituitary LH and plasma follicle-stimulating hormone. **c** Gonadal weight at 71 days in wild-type and hpg males (left) and females (right). Adapted from Cattanach et al. [19].

mRNA (i.e. unable to be translated) encoding the GnRH precursor, thereby preventing GnRH neurons from producing and secreting GnRH. The intimate mechanism was finally unravelled by a Korean team led by K. Kim, who analyzed pre-mRNA GnRH splicing and demonstrated a lack of functional GnRH production, thus explaining the hypogonadotropic hypogonadism of hpg mice [24]. These authors first characterized exonic splicing enhancers located in the two last exons, responsible for activation of first intron splicing [24]. They then demonstrated that genomic deletion of these two last exons led to the accumulation of the intron 1-retained transcripts. When transported to the cytoplasm, these strongly inhibit normal translation of the GnRH peptide by suppressing translational activity of the downstream open reading frame [24].

Normosmic Isolated Congenital Hypogonadotropic Hypogonadism Caused by *GNRH1* Mutations

For many years, we used a candidate gene approach to screen the subgroup of our idiopathic (or isolated) hypogonadotropic hypogonadism (IHH) patients with nonsyndromic and normosmic disease in order to identify mutations in the *GNRH1* gene. After examining nearly 150 unrelated probands, in January 2008 we finally identified a homozygous *GNRH1* frameshift mutation. It consisted of an insertion of an adenine at nucleotide position 18 (c.18–19insA) in the sequence encoding the N-terminal region of the signal peptide-containing protein precursor of GnRH (prepro-GnRH), and was present in two siblings of Romanian origin [25].

The index patient was a young man who was referred at 18 years of age because pubertal development had not occurred. He had typical signs of complete hypogonadism, with small intrascrotal testes, no pubic hair and microphallus, but a normal sense of smell. His affected normosmic sister, who was evaluated at 17 years of age, also had complete hypogonadism, with no breast development, no pubic hair, no menarche, and a small uterus and two small ovaries on ultrasound examination [25]. Both siblings had very low levels of plasma gonadal steroids and serum gonadotropins, a blunted response to GnRH challenge test, normal to low circulating prolactin levels, and otherwise normal pituitary functions. In the sister, who had nonpulsatile baseline LH secretion, we studied the pituitary response to exogenous pulsatile GnRH in order to distinguish between hypothalamic and pituitary gonadotropin deficiency [25, 26]. As was reported by Charlton et al. [27] in the hpg mice, endogenous LH pulsatility was restored by exogenous GnRH administration in this patient, demonstrating the hypothalamic origin of her gonadotropin deficiency and the apparent normal responsiveness of her pituitary gonadotroph cells to GnRH [25–27]. Pulsatile GnRH administration also restored ovarian function, evidenced by increased circulating estradiol and inhibin B levels and the recruitment of a single dominant follicle seen on ultrasound scan. Both index subjects were homozygous for the mutation, whereas their unaffected parents and sister were heterozygous and had a normal reproductive phenotype. The disorder was thus transmitted, as in hpg mice [22], as an autosomal recessive trait. This showed that, in both humans and mice, one copy of both the *GNRH1* and *gnrh1* genes is sufficient for normal GnRH secretion and for normal functioning of the gonadotropic axis, thus ruling out haploinsufficiency [22, 25].

The homozygous mutation in *GNRH1* that we identified in both affected individuals (c.18–19insA) resulted in a frameshift that, if translated, would result in an aberrant peptide starting at amino acid 7 of the GnRH precursor (fig. 3) [25]. This aberrant peptide with a truncated peptide signal sequence devoid of its hydrophobic core was completely deleted of the normal GnRH decapeptide sequence, strongly suggesting its pathological nature; it had a total length of 42 amino acids, instead of the 92 amino acids of the normal prepro-GnRH peptide [25]. In addition, our in vitro experiments clearly demonstrated the deleterious nature of the homozygous mutation, as the transfected *GNRH1* mutant could not sustain GnRH secretion by AtT20 cells (which possess prohormone convertases), while the same cells were capable of producing and secreting mature GnRH when transfected with an expression vector bearing the wild-type *GNRH1* gene [25].

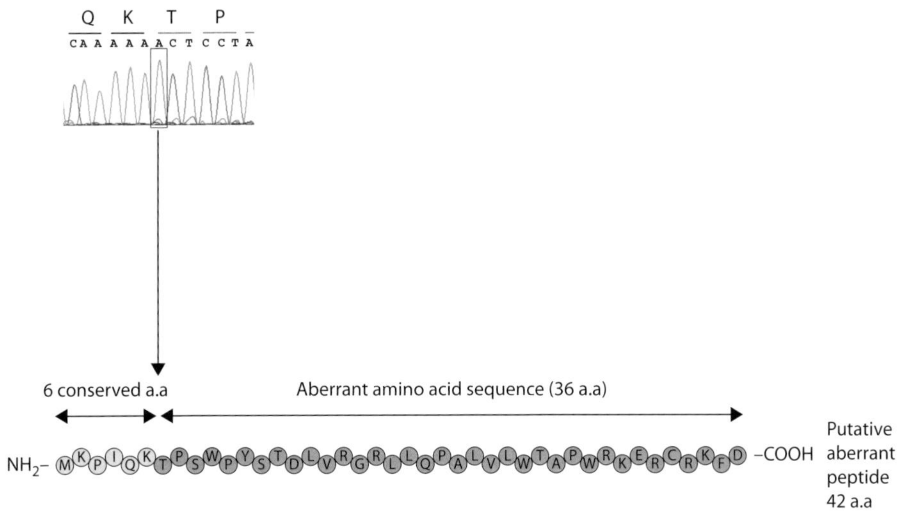

Fig. 3. Homozygous frameshift c.18–19insA *GNRH1* mutation found in 2 patients with isolated normosmic IHH, and its consequences at the peptide level. If translated, this genetic defect would putatively result in an aberrant peptide starting at amino acid 7 with a truncated peptide-signal sequence devoid of its hydrophobic core and a complete lack of the normal GnRH decapeptide sequence. Adapted from Bouligand et al. [25].

It is noteworthy that the 2 IHH subjects had normal to low plasma prolactin levels despite homozygous frameshift mutations, putatively leading to the translation of an aberrant peptide also completely lacking the GAP peptide sequence [25]. Prolactin levels in these 2 patients remained normal despite long-term sex hormone replacement therapy [Ghervan and Young, unpubl. results], excluding the possibility that the normal to low prolactin levels were solely due to sex steroid deficiency [28, 29], and demonstrating that, in physiologic conditions, GAP or putative processed GAP peptides do not act on the human pituitary gland to regulate prolactin secretion, contrary to Seeburg's postulate in his 1985 *Nature* article [12]. In this respect, it is interesting to go back to Cattanach group's first description of the hpg mouse [19]. In their concise and detailed paper, these authors reported a markedly low pituitary prolactin content in both males and females (fig. 4). Oddly, this important finding, which argued strongly against an inhibitory effect of GAP on prolactin secretion, was not alluded to in the paper by Nikolics et al. [12].

Since our first report of a *GNRH1* mutation in IHH, a second homozygous *GNRH1* mutation [(c.87delA/c.87delA)(p.G29GfsX12/p.G29GfsX12)] that was predicted to disrupt the 3 C-terminal amino acids of the GnRH decapeptide and to produce a premature STOP codon was identified in a prepubertal boy originating from Armenia, who was first evaluated at age 8 years and 8 months for cryptorchidism and

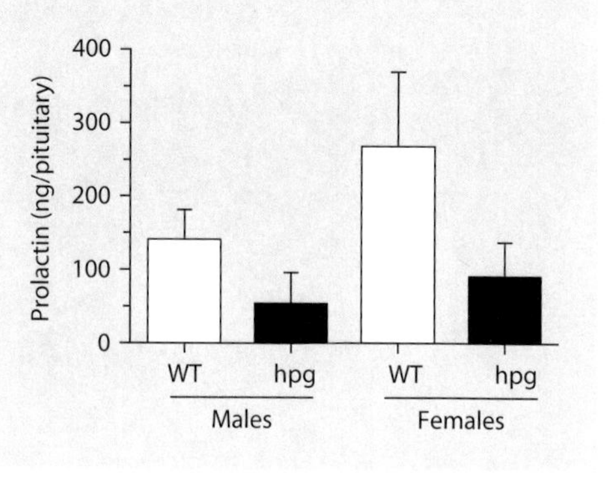

Fig. 4. Pituitary prolactin content in male and female wild-type (WT) and hpg mice. Adapted from Cattanach et al. [19].

microphallus [30]. This child with possible IHH and a normal sense of smell still had no signs of pubertal development at age 13 years 6 months, so he was treated with testosterone enanthate to induce puberty, but was then lost to follow-up. The lack of further clinical or hormonal evaluations means that although IHH was the likeliest diagnosis, simple pubertal delay could not entirely be excluded [31]. Interestingly, the boy's parents, who were most likely heterozygous carriers, had normal pubertal timing, as in the first family we described, further supporting the autosomal recessive transmission of this genetic form of IHH.

In this latter paper, heterozygous variants were also identified in 4 patients with IHH [30], consisting of a nonsynonymous missense mutation of the eighth amino acid of the GnRH decapeptide, a nonsense mutation causing premature termination within GAP, and two sequence variants causing nonsynonymous amino acid substitutions, one in the signal peptide and the other in GAP. However, in the absence of functional data, the contribution of these heterozygous *GNRH1* variants to the pathogenesis of normosmic IHH remains to be established.

References

1 Crowe S, Cushing H, Homans J: Experimental hypophysectomy. Bull Johns Hopkins Hosp 1910;21:127–167.
2 Fink G, Harris GW: The luteinizing hormone releasing activity of extracts of blood from the hypophysial portal vessels of rats. J Physiol 1970;208:221–241.
3 Harris GW: Humours and hormones. J Endocrinol 1972;53:2–23.
4 Raisman G: An urge to explain the incomprehensible: Geoffrey Harris and the discovery of the neural control of the pituitary gland. Annu Rev Neurosci 1997;20:533–566.
5 Matsuo H, Baba Y, Nair RM, Arimura A, Schally AV: Structure of the porcine LH- and FSH-releasing hormone. I. The proposed amino acid sequence. Biochem Biophys Res Commun 1971;43:1334–1339.
6 Amoss M, Burgus R, Blackwell R, Vale W, Fellows R, Guillemin R: Purification, amino acid composition and N-terminus of the hypothalamic luteinizing hormone releasing factor (LRF) of ovine origin. Biochem Biophys Res Commun 1971;44:205–210.

7 Knobil E: The GnRH pulse generator; in Delemarre-van de Waal HA, Plant TM, van Rees GP, Shoemaker J (eds): Control of the Onset of Puberty III. Amsterdam, Elsevier, 1989, pp 11–20.
8 Belchetz PE, Plant TM, Nakai Y, Keogh EJ, Knobil E: Hypophysial responses to continuous and intermittent delivery of hypopthalamic gonadotropin-releasing hormone. Science 1978;202:631–633.
9 Seeburg PH, Adelman JP: Characterization of cDNA for precursor of human luteinizing hormone releasing hormone. Nature 1984;311:666–668.
10 Hayflick JS, Adelman JP, Seeburg PH: The complete nucleotide sequence of the human gonadotropin-releasing hormone gene. Nucleic Acids Res 1989;17: 6403–6404.
11 Adelman JP, Mason AJ, Hayflick JS, Seeburg PH: Isolation of the gene and hypothalamic cDNA for the common precursor of gonadotropin-releasing hormone and prolactin release-inhibiting factor in human and rat. Proc Nat Acad Sci 1986;83:179–183.
12 Nikolics K, Mason AJ, Szonyi E, Ramachandran J, Seeburg PH: A prolactin-inhibiting factor within the precursor for human gonadotropin-releasing hormone. Nature 1985;316:511–517.
13 Yang-Feng TL, Seeburg PH, Francke U: Human luteinizing hormone-releasing hormone gene (LHRH) is located on short arm of chromosome 8 (region 8p11.2-p21). Somat Cell Mol Genet 1986;12: 95–100.
14 Dong KW, Yu KL, Roberts JL: Identification of a major up-stream transcription start site for the human progonadotropin-releasing hormone gene used in reproductive tissues and cell lines. Mol Endocrinol 1993;7:1654–1666.
15 Harris N, Dutlow C, Eidne K, Dong KW, Roberts J, Millar R: Gonadotropin-releasing hormone gene expression in MDA-MB-231 and ZR-75-1 breast carcinoma cell lines. Cancer Res 1991;51:2577–2581.
16 Dong, K-W, Yu KL, Chen ZG, Chen YD, Roberts JL: Characterization of multiple promoters directing tissue-specific expression of the human gonadotropin-releasing hormone gene. Endocrinology 1997; 138:2754–2762.
17 Wolfe A, Kim HH, Tobet S, Stafford DE, Radovick S: Identification of a discrete promoter region of the human GnRH gene that is sufficient for directing neuron-specific expression: a role for POU homeodomain transcription factors. Mol Endocrinol 2002;16:435–449.
18 Chen A, Ganor Y, Rahimipour S, Ben-Aroya N, Koch Y, Levite M: The neuropeptides GnRH-II and GnRH-I are produced by human T cells and trigger laminin receptor gene expression, adhesion, chemotaxis and homing to specific organs. Nat Med 2002; 8:1421–1426.
19 Cattanach BM, Iddon CA, Charlton HM, Chiappa SA, Fink G: Gonadotrophin-releasing hormone deficiency in a mutant mouse with hypogonadism. Nature 1977;269:338–340.
20 Krieger DT, Perlow MJ, Gibson MJ, Davies TF, Zimmerman EA, Ferin M, Charlton HM: Brain grafts reverse hypogonadism of gonadotropin releasing hormone deficiency. Nature 1982;298:468–471.
21 Charlton H: Neural transplantation in hypogonadal (hpg) mice – physiology and neurobiology. Reproduction 2004;127:3–12.
22 Mason AJ, Hayflick JS, Zoeller RT, Young WS III, Phillips HS, Nikolics K, Seeburg PH: A deletion truncating the gonadotropin-releasing hormone gene is responsible for hypogonadism in the hpg mouse. Science 1986;234:1366–1371.
23 Mason AJ, Pitts SL, Nikolics K, Szonyi E, Wilcox JN, Seeburg PH, Stewart TA: The hypogonadal mouse: reproductive functions restored by gene therapy. Science 1986;234:1372–1378.
24 Son GH, Park E, Jung H, Han J, Lee KH, Seong JY, Kim K: GnRH pre-mRNA splicing: solving the mystery of a nature's knockout, hpg mouse. Biochemical and Biophys Res Commun 2005;326:261–267.
25 Bouligand J, Ghervan C, Tello J, Brailly-Tabard S, Salenave S, Chanson P, Lombès M, Millar RM, Guiochon-Mantel A, Young J: Familial isolated hypogonadotropic hypogonadism caused by a mutation in the gonadotropin-releasing hormone gene 1. N Engl J Med 2009;360:2742–748.
26 de Roux N, Young J, Brailly-Tabard S, Misrahi M, Milgrom E, Schaison G: The same molecular defects of the gonadotropin-releasing hormone receptor determine a variable degree of hypogonadism in affected kindred. J Clin Endocrinol Metab 1999;84: 567–572.
27 Charlton HM, Halpin DM, Iddon C, Rosie R, Levy G, McDowell IF, Megson A, Morris JF, Bramwell A, Speight A, Ward BJ, Broadhead J, Davey-Smit G, Fink G: The effects of daily administration of single and multiple injections of gonadotropin-releasing hormone on pituitary and gonadal function in the hypogonadal (hpg) mouse. Endocrinology 1983;113: 535–544.

28 Stanley HF, Curtis A, Sheward WJ, Roberts JL, Fink G: Prolactin messenger ribonucleic acid levels in the normal and hypogonadal mouse pituitary gland. Endocrinology 1986;119:2422–2426.
29 Moshang T Jr, Marx BS, Cara JF, Snyder PJ: The prolactin response to thyrotropin-releasing hormone does not distinguish teenaged males with hypogonadotropic hypogonadism from those with constitutional delay of growth and development. J Clin Endocrinol Metab 1985;61:1211–1213.
30 Chan YM, de Guillebon A, Lang-Muritano M, Plummer L, Cerrato F, Tsiaras S, Gaspert A, Lavoie HB, Wu CH, Crowley WF Jr, Amory JK, Pitteloud N, Seminara SB: GNRH1 mutations in patients with idiopathic hypogonadotropic hypogonadism Proc Natl Acad Sci USA 2009;106:11703–11708.
31 Seminara SB, Hayes FJ, Crowley WE: Gonadotropin-releasing hormone deficiency in the human (idiopathic hypogonadotropic hypogonadism and Kallmann's syndrome): pathophysiological and genetic considerations. Endocr Rev 1998;19:521–539.

Prof. Jacques Young, MD, PhD
Service d'Endocrinologie et des Maladies de la Reproduction
Centre Hospitalier Universitaire de Bicêtre, Assistance Publique Hôpitaux de Paris
78 rue du Général Leclerc, FR–94275 Le Kremlin-Bicêtre Cedex (France)
Tel. +33 1 45213705, Fax +33 1 45212212, E-Mail jacques.young@bct.aphp.fr

Quinton R (ed): Kallmann Syndrome and Hypogonadotropic Hypogonadism.
Front Horm Res. Basel, Karger, 2010, vol 39, pp 121–132

Kallmann Syndrome Caused by Mutations in the *PROK2* and *PROKR2* Genes: Pathophysiology and Genotype-Phenotype Correlations

Julie Sarfati[a,b] · Catherine Dodé[b] · Jacques Young[a,c]

[a]Université Paris-Sud 11 et INSERM U693, Faculté de Médecine Paris Sud, [b]Institut Cochin, INSERM U567, Université René Descartes, [c]Service d'Endocrinologie et des Maladies de la Reproduction, Centre Hospitalier Universitaire de Bicêtre, Assistance Publique Hôpitaux de Paris, Paris, France

Abstract

Mutations in the prokineticin 2 peptide (PROK2) and its seven-transmembrane domain type 2 receptor PROKR2 are newly identified molecular culprits in autosomal Kallmann syndrome (KS). *Prok2* and *prokr2* gene knockout mice both have agenesis or hypoplasia of the olfactory bulbs, associated with hypogonadotropic hypogonadism linked to abnormal GnRH neuron migration. *Prok2–/–* and prokr2–/– mice are the first murine models of this human disease. KS patients of both sexes have a variety of point mutations, missense mutations, frameshifts and nonsense mutations in the *PROK2* and *PROKR2* genes that lead to a loss of peptide or receptor function. When only one allele is affected, penetrance of the two main clinical features of KS may be incomplete: subjects with only one mutant allele may have (1) no symptoms, with normal olfaction and complete pubertal development, (2) congenital isolated (idiopathic) hypogonadotropic hypogonadism (IHH) but normal olfaction, (3) anosmia/hyposmia but normal pubertal development and gonadal function or (4) the two cardinal clinical KS signs, anosmia and IHH. These phenotypic dissociations can be seen in family members with the same *PROK2/PROKR2* mutations. By contrast, patients with two mutant alleles almost always have the cardinal signs of KS. Even when monoallelic *PROK2/PROKR2* mutations are associated with full-blown KS, the reproductive phenotype in males is less severe than in KS associated with biallelic mutations, evidenced by significantly lower frequency of cryptorchidism and micropenis, greater testicular volume, and higher serum levels of LH, FSH and testosterone. Moreover, at least some of these monoallelic cases are in fact digenic, in that they also carry mutations of other KS/IHH genes. Overall, these observations point towards a combination of mendelian autosomal recessive transmission, with more complex oligogenic transmission. Patients with this genetic form of KS have been reported to have a possible increased prevalence of obesity and sleep disorders, which may be related to the role of PROK2 and PROKR2 in food intake and circadian rhythms. However, diurnal variation of serum cortisol levels appears to be physiologically maintained.

A V I T G A **C** D K D S Q **C** G G G M **C** **C** A V S I W V K S
I R I **C** T P M G K L G D S **C** H P L T R K V P F F G R R
M H H T **C** P **C** L P G L A C L R T S F N R F I **C** L A Q K

Fig. 1. Amino acid sequence of human PROK2. The conserved N-terminal hexapeptide is underlined and in bold. The ten conserved cysteine residues are highlighted in bold.

Discovery of the *PROK2* and *PROKR2* Genes

Prokineticins are multifunctional secreted proteins first identified in 2000 by Li et al. [1], who discovered their ability to provoke contraction of smooth muscle fibers in the gastrointestinal tract (hence their name). They were later shown to promote angiogenesis in steroidogenic glands, the heart, and reproductive organs [2]. Their involvement in the Kallmann syndrome (KS) was strongly suggested in 2006 when homozygous Prokr2 knockout mice [3] were shown to have hypogonadotropic hypogonadism due to hypothalamic GnRH deficiency, and agenesis or hypoplasia of the olfactory bulbs. It was confirmed the same year by the discovery of mutations in patients with autosomal KS [4].

PROK2 and Its Receptor PROKR2: Structure, Expression and Actions

In humans, the gene encoding the PROK2 peptide precursor – NCBI Gene ID: 60675; also designated Bv8 to indicate its origin *(Bombina variegata)* and molecular weight (8 kDa) – is located in chromosome region 3p21.1. It has four exons, exon 3 undergoing alternative splicing [5]. The first exon encodes a signal peptide and the first five amino acids, and exons 2 and 3 encode the cysteine-rich domains [5, 6].

The mature form of PROK2 possesses 81 amino acids and shares 40% sequence homology with the related peptide PROK1. As in PROK1, the N-terminal end of PROK2 possesses a sequence of 6 amino acids (AVITGA) (fig. 1) that is fully conserved through evolution and is essential for the peptide's biological activity [6, 7]. Indeed, insertion or deletion of these residues [6, 7] results in peptide antagonism for the receptor. PROK2 also possesses 10 conserved cysteines that participate in the formation of five disulfide bridges with a role in protein folding. Their removal by mutagenesis renders these peptides inactive [6, 7]. Studies of transfected mammalian cells indicate that PROK2 binds with stronger affinity than PROK1 to the PROKR2 receptor, suggesting that it is the main physiological ligand [8, 9]. Prokineticins are expressed in a number of steroidogenic glands, such as the adrenals and testes [10, 11], ovaries [12–13] and placenta [14]. PROK2 is expressed in the central nervous system, where it plays a role in neuron survival by activating the MAP kinase/PI-3-

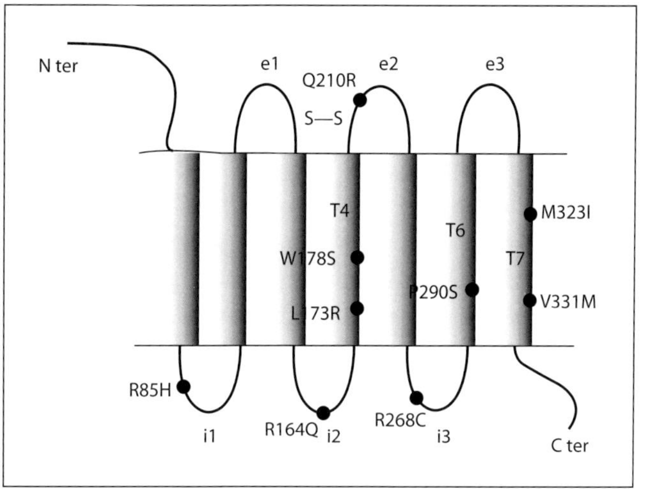

Fig. 2. Schematic representation of the PROKR2 receptor, showing the locations of the nine missense mutations found in familial and nonfamilial cases of KS with respect to the putative N-terminal (N ter), C-terminal (C ter), extracellular loop (e1–e3), intracellular loop (i1–i3), and transmembrane (T1–T7) domains of this G-protein-coupled receptor. Adapted from Dodé et al. [4].

kinase signaling pathway [15]. In the suprachiasmatic nucleus, prok2 transmits the circadian rhythm to the supraoptic nucleus, which is why this signaling pathway is considered to play a key role in the generation of circadian rhythms within the central nervous system [16].

PROKR2, also designated GPR73L1 (NCBI Gene ID: 128674), is a seven-transmembrane domain receptor (fig. 2). Linen et al. [8] mapped the *PROKR2* gene to chromosome region 20p13 in silico. Its transmembrane domains show strong sequence homology with those of PROKR1, which is encoded by a gene lying on a different chromosome [17]. PROKR2 stimulation after transfection of CHO cells provokes calcium release and inositol triphosphate hydrolysis, effects that indicate coupling to a G_q protein. In other cell systems, MAP kinase signaling is inhibited by pertussis toxin, which again suggests coupling to a G_i protein. In mice and humans, respectively, prokr2 and PROKR2 are mainly expressed in the brain [17], the olfactory bulbs [3] and the testes [18]. In the testes, prokineticin-1 is mainly expressed in testosterone-producing Leydig cells, whereas prokineticin-2 expression is restricted to primary spermatocytes [3, 17, 18]. PROK receptors are also expressed in testicular vascular endothelial cells. In the mouse testis, prokr1 and prokr2 are equally expressed, whereas in human testis PROKR1 is expressed more strongly than PROKR2 [3, 17, 18]. The precise roles of each of these ligands and receptors in human testicular physiology remain to be elucidated.

Prok2 and ProkR2 Knockout Mice

In 2005, Ng et al. [19] of the University of California reported the first evidence supporting the involvement of the Prok2/Prokr2 system in olfactory bulb morphogenesis.

The same researchers described the olfactory phenotype of Prok2 knockout mice. They showed that secreted prokineticin 2 functions as a chemoattractant for subventricular zone-derived neuronal progenitors and suggested that, within the olfactory bulbs, prok2 could also act as a detachment signal for chain-migrating progenitors arriving from the rostral migratory stream. Prok2 deficiency in mice leads to a marked reduction in OB size, loss of normal OB architecture, and accumulation of neuronal progenitors within the rostral migratory stream.

As they were focused on the olfactory system, these authors did not describe the gonadotropic phenotype of the knockout mice in their principal study, but a year later, Matsumoto et al. [3] did report a reproductive phenotype resulting from Prokr2 knockout. They showed that *Prokr1–/–* animals had no olfactory bulb defects and a normal reproductive system and, therefore, focused their description on the *Prokr2–/–* animals. They confirmed *Prokr2* expression in the olfactory bulbs of normal mice, which indicated a possible role for this receptor in olfactory bulb morphogenesis. This was subsequently confirmed by the olfactory bulb agenesis observed in *Prokr2–/–* animals. In addition, anatomical analysis showed that both male and female reproductive organ weights were reduced in *Prokr2–/–* mice (but not in Prokr1–/– mice) [3]. No significant differences were observed in the reproductive systems of male and female *Prokr2+/–* heterozygous mice compared with their wild-type counterparts.

Histopathological analysis revealed overt atrophy of the testes and ovaries of all *Prokr2–/–* mice examined. The seminiferous tubules of the latter were reduced in diameter and no sperm were present in the lumen of the tubules in the mutant mice [3]. Spermatogenic cells and spermatocytes were present, but no spermatids were observed. The interstitium was sparse, and very few Leydig cells were observed. Thus, the gonadal phenotype of these animals resembled that of GnRH-lacking hpg mice, pointing to gonadotropin deficiency. Indeed, *Prokr2–/–* mice had all the hormonal characteristics of isolated hypogonadotropic hypogonadism (IHH), namely low levels of pituitary LH and FSH transcripts and low circulating concentrations of these gonadotropins in male mice [3]. The same study indicated that IHH was secondary to GnRH deficiency, based on a clear reduction in the number of GnRH neurons in the preoptic region of the hypothalamus [3]. Thus, *Prokr2–/–* animals had an overall phenotype very similar to that of human patients with the KS.

In 2007, Pitteloud et al. [20] re-analyzed the phenotype of the *Prok2–/–* mice [19] and particularly the reproductive aspects. They showed that *Prok2–/–* mice with olfactory bulb defects did in fact have reproductive abnormalities similar to *Prokr2–/–* mice. Anatomical examination of 12-week-old *Prok2–/–* mice revealed hypoplasia of the reproductive organs in both males and females, with testes and ovaries of *Prok2–/–* mice being significantly smaller than those of age-matched controls. *Prok2–/–* mice exhibited defective GnRH neuron migration, resulting anatomically in a marked decrease in the GnRH neuron population in the hypothalamus and biochemically in IHH [20]. In addition, these authors assessed the gonadal response to gonadotropin stimulation in 4-week-old female *Prok2–/–* mice by giving pregnant mare serum gonadotropin to induce superovulation. These mice could be induced to ovulate after serial injection of gonadotropins and human chorionic gonadotropin, a finding consistent with IHH without any other specific ovarian dysfunction related to prok2 knockout [20].

PROK2 and *PROKR2* Mutations in Kallmann Syndrome

In view of the *Prokr2–/–* mouse phenotype, by 2006 *PROKR2* was considered to be a promising candidate gene for KS [4] and, therefore, the two coding exons of *PROKR2* and the flanking splice sites were sequenced in 192 unrelated KS patients (144 male and 48 female), including 38 familial cases. Ten different mutations (one frameshift and nine missense mutations) were detected in 14 patients (4 familial and 10 apparently sporadic cases). Ten cases were heterozygous, two homozygous and two compound heterozygous.

However, two of these mutations, p.R268C and p.V331M, as well as a mutation (c.253C.T, p.R85C) affecting the same residue as the p.R85H mutation found in 2 KS patients, and another missense mutation (cx1004C.G, p.T335M) not found in the cohort of KS patients, were each detected among 500 alleles from ethnically matched (Caucasian) controls [4]. No other nonsynonymous variants were found in the controls. So even though evidence of conservation of the mutated amino acid residues in bovine, murine and rat orthologous sequences pointed to a deleterious effect of all these missense mutations, without performing functional tests we could not be sure at that time that each missense mutation found in a KS individual was disease causing. Nevertheless, given the KS-like phenotype of Prokr2 knockout mice, the significantly higher overall proportion of *PROKR2* alleles carrying nonsynonymous mutations in KS patients (18 out of 384 alleles) than in controls (4 out of 500 alleles) strongly supported the involvement of this gene in KS [4].

Because PROK2 [8, 9] was thought to be the main ligand of PROKR2, and as mutant mice lacking *Prok2* had atrophic olfactory bulbs with an abnormal architecture, it was also considered possible that mutations in *PROK2* could account for some other cases of KS [4]. Therefore, the four *PROK2* coding exons (including alternatively spliced exon 3 [5, 6] and flanking splice sites) were sequenced in the same cohort of patients. We found four different heterozygous point mutations consisting of two missense mutations, one frameshift (fig. 3) and one single nucleotide substitution in the translation initiation sequence [4] in 2 familial and 2 apparently sporadic cases. These mutations were not detected, and neither were any other variant sequences, in 500 alleles from ethnically matched (Caucasian) control individuals. Interestingly, the p.G32R mutation affected the glycine residue of the highly conserved N-terminal hexapeptide AVITGA (fig. 1) [4, 6, 7]. Since these findings were published, three independent teams [20–23] have found *PROK2* and *PROKR2* mutations, including nonsense mutations [20, 23, 24], further supporting the involvement of these two genes in the pathophysiology of KS. The overall frequency of *PROK2* or *PROKR2*

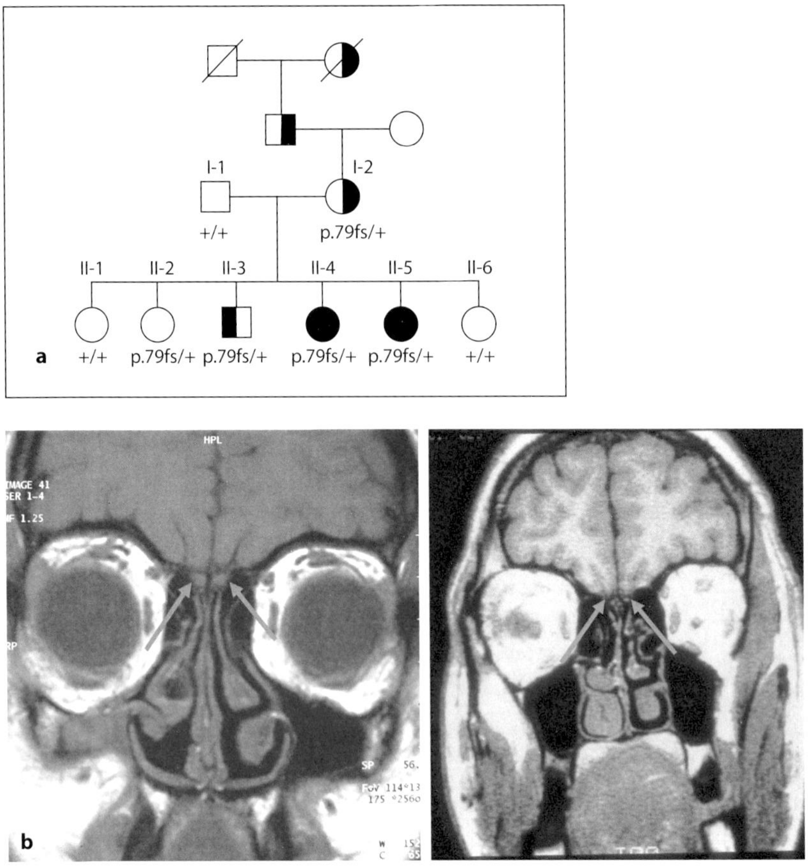

Fig. 3. **a** Segregation of the KS and the PROK2 p.79fsX100 frameshift mutation in an affected family. Half-filled symbols denote individuals with either anosmia only (right half black) or IHH only (left half black). Adapted from Dodé et al. [4]. **b** Normal olfactory bulbs in subject II-3 (arrows, left panel) and olfactory bulb aplasia in subject II-4 (arrows, right panel).

mutations in the combined cohort of more than 600 KS patients is now estimated to be about 9%.

Most KS patients carrying *PROK2* or *PROKR2* point mutations had only one mutated allele. However, as indicated above, a few patients were homozygotes or compound heterozygotes for either *PROK2* or *PROKR2* mutations. This observation, together with both *Prok2* and *Prokr2* knockout mice only exhibiting a KS phenotype in the homozygous state, raises the possibility of digenic transmission of the human disease in heterozygous patients, i.e. affected individuals harboring heterozygous *PROK2* or *PROKR2* mutations possibly only have KS because they harbor mutation(s) of other gene(s) as well. However, so far, this has been confirmed in only a few patients carrying missense mutations in both *PROKR2* and *KAL1*, or in *PROKR2* and *PROK2* [4, 23, 25], suggesting that the putative second mutation in heterozygous patients might lie in unexplored regions of the genes or in as yet undiscovered KS culprit genes. An alternative possibility is that some PROKR2 missense mutations could have a dominant negative effect on the normal allele, but this mechanism is unlikely to account for the deleterious effect of all missense mutations, as many of these mutations have also been found in somatically and reproductively normal individuals [20–24].

***PROK2* and *PROKR2* Mutations in Kallmann Syndrome Are Loss-of-Function Mutations**

This was predicted by the phenotype of *Prok2–/–* and *Prokr2–/–* mice, and was also strongly suggested by the existence of nonsense mutations putatively generating truncated proteins [4, 20, 21, 23, 24]. However, the first formal demonstration of loss of PROK2 function induced by a natural human *PROK2* mutation was reported by Pitteloud et al. [20] and Cole et al. [21]. These authors investigated the bioactivity of a number of natural mutant proteins in vitro. Specifically, they examined the signaling properties of four PROK2 mutants (C34Y, I50M, R73C and I55X) in an aequorin-based luminescence assay of intracellular calcium mobilization. They showed first that the full-length human PROK2 (hPROK2) activated PROKR2 at low concentrations (EC50 ~50 nM) and, second, that the C34Y mutation totally abolished the calcium-mobilizing activity of PROK2. The R73C mutation resulted in a 7-fold decrease in activity at the wild-type EC50. The truncated PROK2–27AA (p.I55fsX1) could not activate PROKR2 even at very high concentrations [20, 21]. In addition, these authors assessed the functionality of the PROKR2 mutant in an Egr1-LUC gene transcription assay as well as in an aequorin-based Ca^{2+} flux assay. They demonstrated that, in both systems, the wild-type receptor yielded dose-response curves with 10- to 15-fold and 40- to 50-fold maximum induction, respectively, whereas the six PROKR2 mutants (Y113H, V115M, R164Q, L173R, W178S and S188L) showed severely altered activity in both assays. Furthermore, all the mutants showed markedly reduced expression, suggesting that protein instability may in part explain their poor biological function [21].

In a recent paper, Monnier et al. [26] also showed that PROKR2 missense mutations associated with KS impair receptor signaling activity. These authors studied ten different missense natural mutations (p.R85C, p.R85H, p.R164Q, p.L173R, p.W178S, p.Q210R, p.R268C, p.P290S, p.M323I, p.V331M) that were identified in PROKR2. They reproduced each of the ten mutations in a recombinant murine Prokr2, and tested their effects on the signaling activity in transfected HEK-293 cells by measuring intracellular calcium release upon ligand-activation of the receptor. They found that all mutated receptors except one (M323I) had reduced signaling activity. Three mutations (L173R, W178S, P290S) impaired cell surface targeting of the receptor, one mutation (Q210R) abolished ligand binding, and five mutations (R85C, R85H, R164Q, R268C, V331M) were presumed to impair G-protein coupling of the receptor. In addition, when wild-type and mutant receptors were coexpressed in HEK-293

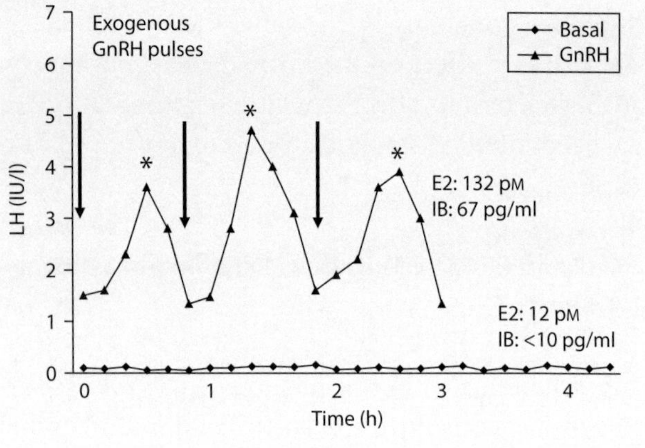

Fig. 4. Baseline LH secretion in a 22-year-old woman (subject II-4; fig. 3a) carrying a p.79fsX100 frameshift mutation in *PROK2*. LH secretion was also evaluated on day 22 of pulsatile GnRH administration, as described in Salenave et al. [30]. Arrows indicate exogenous GnRH boluses (10 μg) and asterisks denote detectable LH pulses. E2 = Plasma estradiol level; IB = serum inhibin B level.

cells, none of the mutant receptors that were retained within the cells affected cell surface targeting of the wild-type receptor, and none of the mutant receptors properly addressed at the plasma membrane affected wild-type receptor signaling activity. These results argue against a dominant negative effect of the mutations in vivo, and are congruent with the lack of phenotypic defects in some heterozygous carriers.

Genotype-Phenotype Correlations

PROK2 and *PROKR2* mutations mainly give rise to a phenotype that includes both IHH and anosmia or hyposmia, with a low prevalence of other non-reproductive phenotypes [4, 20–25]. With regard to IHH, the response to pulsatile GnRH administration (fig. 4) points to hypothalamic involvement. This suggests that, as reported in prok2–/– and *Prokr2–/–* rodents (and shown many years ago in a fetus with a *KAL1* abnormality), mutations of factors involved in PROK2/PROKR2 signaling could affect the migration of GnRH neurons in humans. However, as was already shown in kindreds harboring heterozygous *FGFR1* loss-of-function mutations [27–30], some carriers of *PROK2* or *PROKR2* loss-of-function mutations within a given family can have isolated IHH, isolated anosmia, or even be asymptomatic. A definitive explanation for this may have to await the day when all potential IHH-causing genes are known, enabling family members to be screened for these systematically. It is noteworthy that normal phenotype is most often associated with monoallelic *PROK2/PROKR2* mutations (fig. 3), whereas most individuals with two mutated alleles are markedly affected [4, 20–25]. Forms that are partially reversible on treatment have also been described [21, 22].

We recently studied 55 adult KS patients (42 men and 13 women) carrying mutations in *PROK2* or *PROKR2*, comprising 41 monoallelic and 14 biallelic cases [25].

Table 1. Clinical features reported in subjects carrying *PROK2/PROKR2* mutations

Clinical feature	*PROK2* mutations	*PROKR2* mutations	References
Normal puberty	yes*	yes*	[4, 20–24, 25]
IHH	yes	yes	[4, 20–24, 25]
Normal sense of smell	yes*	yes*	[4, 20–24]
Anosmia/hyposmia	yes	yes	[4, 20–24, 25]
Cleft lip/palate, high-arched palate	yes*	yes*	[23, 25]
Dental agenesis	no	yes*	[25]
Hearing loss	yes*	yes*	[21, 25]
Ptosis/ocular nerve conduction disorders	no	no	–
Bimanual synkinesia	yes*	yes*	[21, 25]
Epilepsy	yes	yes	[20, 21]
Sleep disorders	yes	yes	[4, 21]
Overweight or obesity	yes	yes	[4, 23]
Cryptorchidism	yes	yes	[21, 23, 25]
Other genital anomaly (vas deferens aplasia, etc.)	no	no	–
Renal anomaly (agenesis, horseshoe kidney, etc.)	no	no	[25]
Bone abnormalities	yes	yes	[20, 21]

Asterisk signifies only in subjects with heterozygous mutations.

Biallelic mutations were associated with a significantly more severe reproductive phenotype in males, with greater frequency of cryptorchidism (70 vs. 34%), and micropenis (90 vs. 28%), lower testicular volume (1.2 vs. 4.5 ml), lower basal serum FSH (0.3 vs. 1.8 IU/l) and testosterone (0.2 vs. 0.7 ng/ml) levels, and weaker LH response to GnRH-stimulation (0.8 vs. 5.2 IU/l). Table 1 shows the main manifestations of KS [31–33] in subjects with *PROK2/PROKR2* mutations. In addition to IHH and anosmia/hyposmia, some non-reproductive abnormalities described in other genetic forms of KS are also seen, such as mirror movements (synkinesis) and congenital ptosis, but no cases of renal agenesis or malformation have been reported [20–25]. Apart from anosmia, the non-reproductive defects seem to be restricted to patients with monoallelic mutations. However, in our recent study [25], five of 41 'monoallelic' *PROK2/PROKR2* cases were, in fact, found to be digenic in that they also harbored mutations of other IHH/KS genes (*KAL1* ×2, *FGFR1*, *GHRHR* and *GPR54/KISSR*). It thus remains possible that the remaining 36 cases will eventually be found to harbor mutations of other genes that have yet to be identified. Our working hypothesis is that biallelic (homozygous and compound heterozygous) *PROK2* and *PROKR2* mutations can themselves cause IHH, with or without anosmia, but rarely any other non-reproductive anomaly. By contrast, heterozygous *PROK2* and *PROKR2* mutations may only be able to cause significant reproductive (and non-reproductive) phenotypes when combined with mutations of another IHH/KS gene.

Specific sleep disorders appear to exist too, but no precise comparative studies of patients with *PROK2/PROKR2* mutations with other genetic forms of KS have been conducted in order to confirm the presence of circadian disorders similar to those described in *prok2/prokr2* rodents [16, 34]. Physiological diurnal variation of serum cortisol levels appears to be preserved [25], but there is a suggestion that mood disorder may be more prevalent among *PROKR2* mutation carriers than in the general (Japanese) population [35].

The gonadal expression of prokineticins and their receptors suggests that PROK2 or PROKR2 mutations could potentially lead to ovarian or testicular disorders independent of gonadotropin deficiency. A phenomenon of this type has been described in the testes of mice and patients with *Dax1* knock-out and *DAX1* loss-of-function mutations, respectively [36, 37]. However, anecdotal data indicate that spermatogenesis and ovulation are not more difficult to induce in IHH subjects with *PROK2/PROKR2* mutations [20], but larger studies are needed to confirm this.

Because the PROK/PROKR2 system has been linked to obesity in rodents [38] – in particular, activation of this system results in an anorexigenic response – the body mass index has been analyzed in some KS patients. Dodé et al. [4] reported the case of a KS patient heterozygous for the p.R73C mutation of *PROK2*, who was markedly overweight and had severe sleep disorder. Abreu et al. [23] reported that 3 of 5 KS patients with *PROKR2* mutations were obese and that a 50-year-old woman heterozygous for the p.L173R mutation had the metabolic syndrome. Here again, however, the body mass index needs to be studied systematically in the different genetic forms of KS and related disorders, and compared with the reference population, before concluding that this genetic form is associated with hyperphagia and/or obesity.

References

1 Li M, Bullock CM, Knauer DJ, Ehlert FJ, Zhou QY: Identification of two prokineticin cDNAs: recombinant proteins potently contract gastrointestinal smooth muscle. Mol Pharmacol 2001;59:692–698.

2 LeCouter J, Kowalski J, Foster J, Hass P, Zhang Z, Dillard-Telm L, Frantz G, Rangell L, DeGuzman L, Keller GA, Peale F, Gurney A, Hillan KJ, Ferrara N: Identification of an angiogenic mitogen selective for endocrine gland endothelium. Nature 2001;412:877–884.

3 Matsumoto S, Yamazaki C, Masumoto KH, et al: Abnormal development of the olfactory bulb and reproductive system in mice lacking prokineticin receptor PKR2. Proc Natl Acad Sci USA 2006;103:4140–4145.

4 Dodé C, Teixeira L, Levilliers J, et al: Kallmann syndrome: mutations in the genes encoding prokineticin-2 and prokineticin receptor-2. PLoS Genet 2006;2:e175.

5 Jilek A, Engel E, Beier D, Lepperdinger G: Murine Bv8 gene maps near a synteny breakpoint of mouse chromosome 6 and human 3p21. Gene 2000;256:189–195.

6 Bullock CM, Li JD, Zhou QY: Structural determinants required for the bioactivities of prokineticins and identification of prokineticin receptor antagonists. Mol Pharmacol 2004;65:582–588.

7 Negri L, Lattanzi R, Giannini E, Melchiorri P: Bv8/Prokineticin proteins and their receptors. Life Sci 2007;81:1103–1116.

8 Lin DC, Bullock CM, Ehlert FJ, Chen JL, Tian H, Zhou QY: Identification and molecular characterization of two closely related G protein-coupled receptors activated by prokineticins/endocrine gland vascular endothelial growth factor. J Biol Chem 2002;277:19276–19280.

9 Masuda Y, Takatsu Y, Terao Y, Kumano S, Ishibashi Y, Suenaga M, Abe M, Fukusumi S, Watanabe T, Shintani Y, Yamada T, Hinuma S, Inatomi N, Ohtaki T, Onda H, Fujino M: Isolation and identification of EG-VEGF/prokineticins as cognate ligands for two orphan G-protein-coupled receptors. Biochem Biophys Res Commun 2002;293:396–402.

10 Maldonado-Pérez D, Evans J, Denison F, Millar RP, Jabbour HN: Potential roles of the prokineticins in reproduction. Trends Endocrinol Metab 2007;18:66–72.

11 LeCouter J, Lin R, Tejada M, Frantz G, Peale F, Hillan KJ, Ferrara N: The endocrine-gland-derived VEGF homologue Bv8 promotes angiogenesis in the testis: localization of Bv8 receptors to endothelial cells. Proc Natl Acad Sci USA 2003;100:2685–2690.

12 Ferrara N, Frantz G, LeCouter J, Dillard-Telm L, Pham T, Draksharapu A, Giordano T, Peale F: Differential expression of the angiogenic factor genes vascular endothelial growth factor (VEGF) and endocrine gland-derived VEGF in normal and polycystic human ovaries. Am J Pathol 2003;162: 1881–1893.

13 Fraser HM, Bell J, Wilson H, Taylor PD, Morgan K, Anderson RA, Duncan WC: Localization and quantification of cyclic changes in the expression of endocrine gland vascular endothelial growth factor in the human corpus luteum. J Clin Endocrinol Metab 2005;90:427–434.

14 Hoffmann P, Feige JJ, Alfaidy N: Expression and oxygen regulation of endocrine gland-derived vascular endothelial growth factor/prokineticin-1 and its receptors in human placenta during early pregnancy. Endocrinology 2006;147:1675–1684.

15 Lin R, LeCouter J, Kowalski J, Ferrara N: Characterization of endocrine gland-derived vascular endothelial growth factor signaling in adrenal cortex capillary endothelial cells. J Biol Chem 2002; 277:8724–8729.

16 Cheng MY, Bullock CM, Li C, Lee AG, Bermak JC, Belluzzi J, Weaver DR, Leslie FM, Zhou QY: Prokineticin 2 transmits the behavioural circadian rhythm of the suprachiasmatic nucleus. Nature 2002;417:405–410.

17 Soga T, Matsumoto S, Oda T, Saito T, Hiyama H, Takasaki J, Kamohara M, Ohishi T, Matsushime H, Furuichi K: Molecular cloning and characterization of prokineticin receptors. Biochim Biophys Acta 2002;1579:173–179.

18 Wechselberger C, Puglisi R, Engel E, Lepperdinger G, Boitani C, Kreil G: The mammalian homologues of frog Bv8 are mainly expressed in spermatocytes. FEBS Lett 1999;462:177–181.

19 Ng KL, Li JD, Cheng MY, Leslie FM, Lee AG, Zhou QY: Dependence of olfactory bulb neurogenesis on prokineticin 2 signaling. Science 2005;308:1923–1927.

20 Pitteloud N, Zhang C, Pignatelli D, Li JD, Raivio T, Cole LW, Plummer L, Jacobson-Dickman EE, Mellon PL, Zhou QY, Crowley WF Jr: Loss-of-function mutation in the prokineticin 2 gene causes Kallmann syndrome and normosmic idiopathic hypogonadotropic hypogonadism. Proc Natl Acad Sci USA 2007;104:17447–17452.

21 Cole LW, Sidis Y, Zhang C, et al: Mutations in prokineticin 2 and prokineticin receptor 2 genes in human gonadotrophin-releasing hormone deficiency: molecular genetics and clinical spectrum. J Clin Endocrinol Metab 2008;93:3551–3559.

22 Sinisi AA, Asci R, Bellastella G, Maione L, Esposito D, Elefante A, De Bellis A, Bellastella A, Iolascon A: Homozygous mutation in the prokineticin-receptor 2 gene (Val274Asp) presenting as reversible Kallmann syndrome and persistent oligozoospermia: case report. Hum Reprod 2008;23:2380–2384.

23 Abreu AP, Trarbach EB, de Castro M, Costa EM, Versiani B, Baptista MT, Garmes HM, Mendonca BB, Latronico AC: Loss-of-function mutations in the genes encoding prokineticin-2 or prokineticin-receptor-2 cause autosomal recessive Kallmann syndrome. J Clin Endocrinol Metab 2008;93:4113–4118.

24 Leroy C, Fouveaut C, Leclercq S, Jacquemont S, Boullay HD, Lespinasse J, Delpech M, Dupont JM, Hardelin JP, Dodé C: Biallelic mutations in the prokineticin-2 gene in two sporadic cases of Kallmann syndrome. Eur J Hum Genet 2008;16:865–868.

25 Sarfati J, Guiochon-Mantel A, Rondard P, et al: A comparative phenotypic study of Kallmann syndrome patients carrying monoallelic and biallelic mutations in the prokineticin 2 (PROK2) or prokineticin receptor 2 (PROKR2) genes. J Clin Endocrinol Metab 2010, Epub ahead of print.

26 Monnier C, Dodé C, Fabre L, Teixeira L, Labesse G, Pin JP, Hardelin JP, Rondard P: PROKR2 missense mutations associated with Kallmann syndrome impair receptor signalling-activity. Hum Mol Genet 2009;18:75–81.

27 Dodé C, Levilliers J, Dupont JM, et al: Loss-of-function mutations in FGFR1 cause autosomal dominant Kallmann syndrome. Nat Genet 2003;33: 463–465.

28 Albuisson J, Pêcheux C, Carel JC, Lacombe D, Leheup B, Lapuzina P, Bouchard P, Legius E, Matthijs G, Wasniewska M, Delpech M, Young J, Hardelin JP, Dodé C: Kallmann syndrome: 14 novel mutations in KAL1 and FGFR1 (KAL2). Hum Mutat 2005;25:98–109.

29 Dodé C, Fouveaut C, Mortier G, Janssens S, Bertherat J, Mahoudeau J, Kottler ML, Chabrolle C, Gancel A, François I, Devriendt K, Wolczynski S, Pugeat M, Pineiro-Garcia A, Murat A, Bouchard P, Young J, Delpech M, Hardelin JP: Novel FGFR1 sequence variants in Kallmann syndrome, and genetic evidence that the FGFR1c isoform is required in olfactory bulb and palate morphogenesis. Hum Mutat 2007;28:97–108.
30 Salenave S, Chanson P, Bry H, Pugeat M, Cabrol S, Carel JC, Murat A, Lecomte P, Brailly S, Hardelin JP, Dodé C, Young J: Kallmann's syndrome: a comparison of the reproductive phenotypes in men carrying KAL1 and FGFR1/KAL2 mutations. J Clin Endocrinol Metab 2008;93:758–763.
31 Hardelin JP: Kallmann syndrome: towards molecular pathogenesis. Mol Cell Endocrinol 2001;179:75–81.
32 Dodé C, Hardelin JP: Kallmann syndrome: fibroblast growth factor signaling insufficiency? J Mol Med 2004;82:725–734.
33 Hardelin JP, Petit C: A molecular approach to the pathophysiology of the X chromosome-linked Kallmann's syndrome. Baillieres Clin Endocrinol Metab 1995;9:489–507.
34 Hu WP, Li JD, Zhang C, Boehmer L, Siegel JM, Zhou QY: Altered circadian and homeostatic sleep regulation in prokineticin 2-deficient mice. Sleep 2007;30:247–256.
35 Kishi T, Kitajima T, Tsunoka T, Okomura T, Ikeda M, Okochi T, Kinoshita Y, Kawashima K, Yamanouchi Y, Ozaki N, Iwata N: Possible association of prokineticin 2 receptor gene (PROK2) with mood disorders in the Japanese population. Neuromolecular Med 2009;11:114–122.
36 Caron P, Imbeaud S, Bennet A, Plantavid M, Camerino G, Rochiccioli P: Combined hypothalamic-pituitary-gonadal defect in a hypogonadic man with a novel mutation in the DAX-1 gene. J Clin Endocrinol Metab 1999;84:3563–3569.
37 Tabarin A, Achermann JC, Recan D, Bex V, Bertagna X, Christin-Maitre S, Ito M, Jameson JL, Bouchard P: A novel mutation in DAX1 causes delayed-onset adrenal insufficiency and incomplete hypogonadotropic hypogonadism. J Clin Invest 2000;105:321–328.
38 Negri L, Lattanzi R, Giannini E, De Felice M, Colucci A, Melchiorri P: Bv8, the amphibian homologue of the mammalian prokineticins, modulates ingestive behaviour in rats. Br J Pharmacol 2004;142:181–191.

Prof. Jacques Young, MD, PhD
Service d'Endocrinologie et des Maladies de la Reproduction
Centre Hospitalier Universitaire de Bicêtre, Assistance Publique Hôpitaux de Paris
78 rue du Général Leclerc, FR–94275 Le Kremlin-Bicêtre Cedex (France)
Tel. +33 1 45213705, Fax +33 1 45212212, E-Mail jacques.young@bct.aphp.fr

Quinton R (ed): Kallmann Syndrome and Hypogonadotropic Hypogonadism.
Front Horm Res. Basel, Karger, 2010, vol 39, pp 133–141

Neurokinin B and Its Receptor in Hypogonadotropic Hypogonadism

Robert K. Semple[a] · A. Kemal Topaloglu[b]

[a]University of Cambridge Metabolic Research Laboratories, Institute of Metabolic Science, Addenbrooke's Hospital, Cambridge, UK; [b]Department of Pediatric Endocrinology and Metabolism, Faculty of Medicine, Cukurova University, Adana, Turkey

Abstract

The hypothalamus integrates multiple environmental and developmental cues relevant to reproductive function, serving to transduce these into a pulsatile output of gonadotropin-releasing hormone (GnRH). Although neuroanatomical and physiological studies have yielded key clues about the functional organisation of the so-called 'GnRH pulse generator', only in the last decade have the molecular components of the circuitry upstream from GnRH begun to be elucidated. A major contributor to this has been human genetics, through identification of mutations causing isolated hypogonadotropic hypogonadism (IHH) without developmental defects. The greatest success of this approach was the finding in 2003 that mutations of *KISS1R* cause IHH, producing a quantum leap in understanding of regulation of GnRH secretion, and energising the field. New evidence has now emerged that loss of function of neurokinin B (NKB) or its receptor, the neurokinin-3 receptor, produces IHH of similar severity to that caused by *KISS1R* mutations in humans. Preliminary evidence suggests that the role of NKB in reproductive function differs significantly between humans and rodents, posing challenges for future studies. We review the human genetics of NKB and its receptor, and discuss the future work required to elucidate their precise role in the regulation of human GnRH secretion.

Improved understanding of the development and regulation of the human gonadotropin-releasing hormone (GnRH) pulse generator will be essential in order to elucidate the pathogenesis of disorders of sexual maturation, to improve manipulation of human reproductive and gonadal endocrine function for therapeutic benefit, and to answer fundamental questions about the timing of puberty. The quest to achieve understanding at cellular and molecular resolution of the human hypothalamic-pituitary-gonadal (HPG) axis has been a long one, but one that has been excitingly illuminated in recent years by an increasing rate of discovery of human genetic disorders directly affecting HPG axis ontogeny and/or function [1].

Of most relevance to the regulation of the function of anatomically normal GnRH neurones, and thus most likely to yield clear therapeutic targets in human disease, are those defects which produce pure isolated hypogonadotropic hypogonadism (IHH) without anosmia, other developmental defects, or other hormonal deficits – that is, normosmic IHH (nIHH). It is in this area that human genetics has made a particularly large contribution over the past decade, most notably through the quantum leap in understanding of the regulation of GnRH secretion stimulated by genetic demonstration that loss of KISS1R function produces nIHH [2, 3]. Excitingly from a scientific point of view, only a minority of cases of nIHH are accounted for by mutations in *KISS1R*, *GNRHR* or *GNRH1*, the last two named encoding the GnRH/GnRHR ligand receptor pair, suggesting that human 'experiments of nature' still have much valuable information to yield about human HPG function [1, 4].

Identification of *TACR3* and *TAC3* Mutations in Normosmic Isolated Hypogonadotropic Hypogonadism

For this reason, we recently set out to identify new genetic causes of nIHH by focussing on consanguineous families with more than one member affected by nIHH [5]. In each case, mutations in *GNRH1, GNRHR, KISS1, KISS1R* among others were excluded prior to genome-wide typing of single nucleotide polymorphisms using genomic microarrays. Using prevalence data for each nucleotide variant, it was possible to compute which areas of the genome in each individual were homozygous. These areas of homozygosity were aligned for all family members, and a search was conducted for areas that were homozygous in all affected, but no unaffected individuals, based on the assumption that the hormonal deficit was caused by homozygosity for an autosomal recessive mutation.

The results from the application of this approach to ten families were striking: in four families, heavily overlapping short segments of chromosome 4 were implicated, containing only around twenty known or predicted genes [5, 6]. Of these, *TACR3*, encoding the G_q-coupled neurokinin 3 receptor, which is the endogenous receptor for neurokinin B (NKB), was the most obvious candidate based on prior animal studies (which will be described later). Sequencing of *TACR3* in all families revealed three different homozygous mutations of conserved residues, one of which – Pro353Ser – was found in two families (fig. 1). When studied in cell culture, all mutants had severely reduced ability to mediate a rise in cytosolic calcium in response to NKB (fig. 1) [5, 6].

In light of these findings, genotyping results in other families were reviewed. In one of these, a relatively large area of chromosome 12 was implicated in causing nIHH. Although this encoded a daunting 102 known or predicted genes, *TAC3*, encoding NKB, was amongst them. On sequencing this family, a homozygous mutation was found substituting the exquisitely conserved terminal methionine of the mature

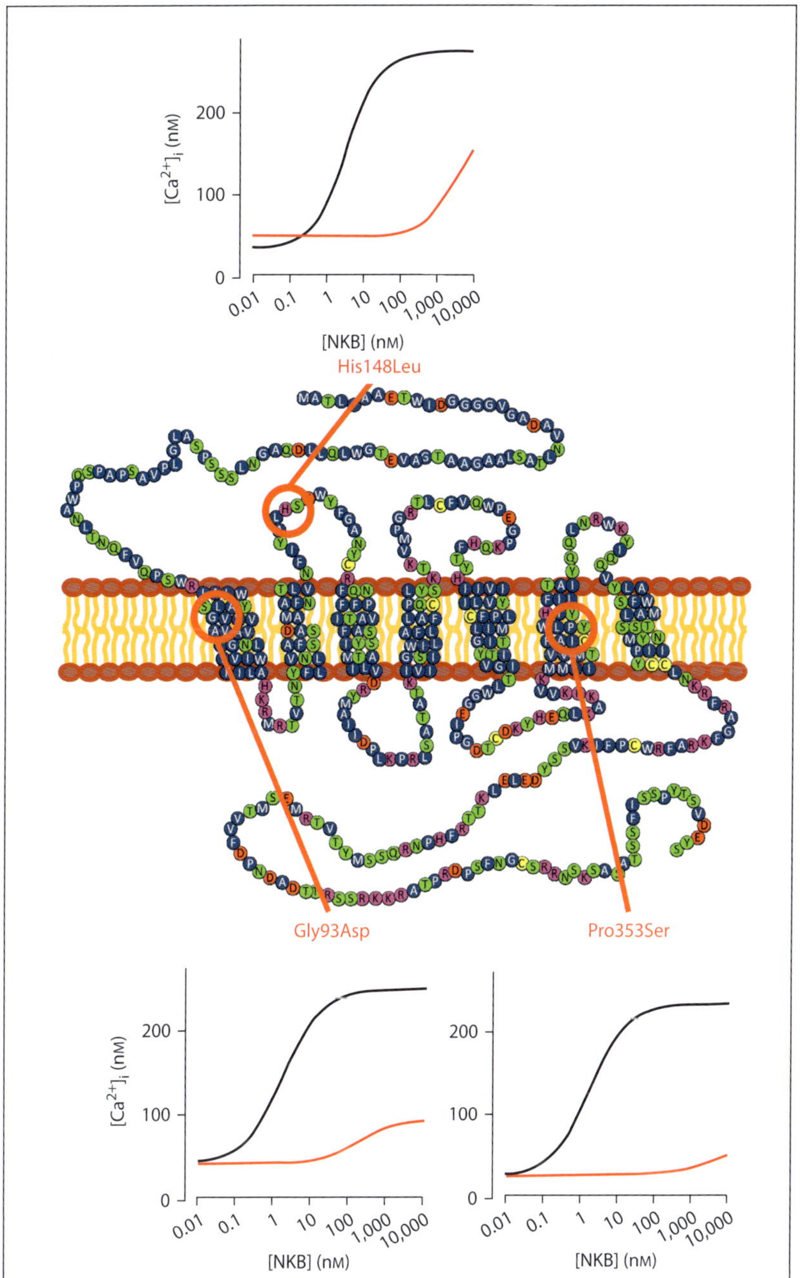

Fig. 1. Schematic of the neurokinin 3 receptor with location of homozygous missense mutations described in association with HH. For each mutation, calcium flux in response to wild-type NKB is shown in red, relative to the response of the wild-type receptor in black.

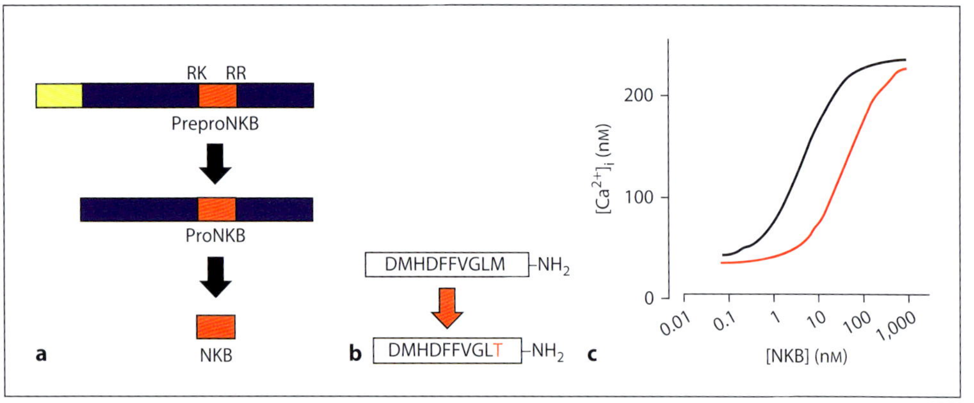

Fig. 2. Site and functional consequence of homozygous missense mutation in NKB. **a** Processing of NKB precursors to yield mature NKB. **b** Site of mutated methionine (in red) in patients with nIHH. **c** Reduction in ability of mutant NKB (in red) to elicit calcium flux at the wild-type neurokinin 3 receptor compared to wild-type NKB (in black).

neuropeptide to threonine [5]. In endogenous NKB, this terminal methionine is amidated. Although it is not possible to be certain that the threonine introduced at the same position of the mutant NKB is also amidated in vivo, a single enzyme in humans is responsible for all peptide C-terminal amidations, and is relatively insensitive to primary structure at the amidation site [7], and so it seems most likely that in affected humans the threonine-containing peptide is also amidated. In vitro, non-amidated mutant NKB had no significant ability to stimulate the wild-type NK3R, while amidated mutant NKB had an EC_{50} around 10-fold lower than wild-type NKB (fig. 2) [5].

Thus, a total of five out of ten consanguineous families with familial, autosomal recessive nIHH harboured loss-of-function mutations in either the gene encoding NKB or its receptor, firmly establishing that intact NKB/NK3R function is necessary for normal human HPG function. It remains to be determined in larger studies how prevalent such mutations are in nIHH on more diverse ethnic backgrounds. However, although all the families studied to date originated from Turkey, three different receptor mutations and one ligand mutation were found, suggesting that this apparently high local prevalence does not represent a geographic founder effect. On the other hand, 50 sporadic cases of nIHH from the same region were found not to have either *TACR3* or *TAC3* mutations.

Phenotypes of Patients with *TACR3* or *TAC3* Mutations

A summary of the clinical and endocrine features of affected patients is shown in table 1. All affected patients had unequivocal and profound IHH, including some individuals in their mid 20s. Affected males all had microphallus and cryptorchidism,

Table 1. Clinical, genetic and biochemical features of patients with loss-of-function mutations in *TAC3* or *TACR3*

	Family										
	1		2		3		4			5	
Sex	F	M	M	F	F	F	F	M	M	F	F
Age, years	20	24	12.8	15.3	16.2	14	26	25	14.5	21.5	17.5
Pathogenic mutation	*TACR3* G93D	*TACR3* G93D	*TACR3* P353S	*TACR3* P353S	*TACR3* P353S	*TACR3* P353S	*TACR3* H148L	*TACR3* H148L	*TACR3* H148L	*TAC3* M90T	*TAC3* M90T
Tanner stage	B1P3	G1P3	G1P3	B1P3	B1P3	B1P3	B1P1	G1P1	G1P1	B1P2	B1P2
Other clinical features	PA	MP	MP; CO	PA	PA	PA	PA	MP	MP; CO	PA; ↓ IQ	PA; ↓ IQ
LH, U/l	0.1	0.2	0.1	0.5	0.3	0.1	0.1	2.7	0.1	0.06	0.1
FSH, U/l	3.2	3.0	1.2	4.9	2.1	2.0	0.9	5.3	0.7	0.05	0.41
E_2, pM	9.5	–	–	1.9	3.7	1.9	0.6	–	–	0.4	<0.1
Testosterone, nM	–	0.4	0.4	–	–	–	–	2.4	<0.1	–	–
GnRH stimulation test											
Peak FSH, U/l	12.8	11.5	6.4	16.3	8.0	8.5	11.0	–	2.9	2.2	2.2
Peak LH, U/l	2.9	3.2	2.3	6.2	2.3	0.9	4.0	–	0.5	2.5	3.8

MP = Microphallus; CO = cryptorchidism; PA = primary amenorrhoea.

suggesting that NKB and its receptor are necessary for appropriate intrauterine HPG activation as well as being required for later sexual maturation at puberty. In no case was there any clinical evidence of developmental abnormalities such as anosmia, cleft lip or palate, retinitis pigmentosa, iris colobomata, hearing loss, or hypotonia. However, the 2 siblings with *TAC3* mutations had mild cognitive impairment with poor educational attainment, at odds with their unaffected siblings, and with all the patients with homozygous *TACR3* mutations. While it cannot be concluded based on two siblings from a single consanguineous family that cognitive impairment is a general feature of *TAC3* mutations, it does raise the possibility that loss of NKB may have more widespread consequences than loss of the NK3R, perhaps reflecting some action of NKB at other receptors such as the NK1R and NK2R. This would be in line with data implicating NKB in a variety of cognitive processes and disorders [8–13]. No patient with *TACR3* or *TAC3* mutations has yet sought to conceive, and so it remains unclear whether maternal TAC3/TACR3 play any non-redundant role in placental function, a possibility raised by expression of NKB in human syncytiotrophoblast and by the elevated levels of circulating NKB seen in human pregnancy [14, 15].

Role of Neurokinin B in Reproductive Function

Neurokinins belong to the tachykinin family of signalling peptides, a phylogenetically ancient group with widespread signalling roles in both vertebrates and invertebrates [16]. In humans, the best known tachykinins are substance P (SP) and neurokinin A (NKA) – different peptide products of the same gene, *TAC1* – and NKB. All are widely expressed in the CNS, and SP and NKA are believed predominantly to function in nociception [16]. The dominant function of NKB has not been clearly appreciated before now. Although widely expressed in the CNS in both humans and rodents, both *TAC3* and *TACR3* are expressed peripherally in placenta, kidney, skeletal muscle and lung among other tissues [17]. A significant body of work has implicated NKB in diverse functions, including water homeostasis [18], pulmonary inflammation [19], and cognition [8, 9].

Prior to the human genetic discovery of loss of function mutations, there had also been a growing body of work in animal models building a case for an important role in regulating reproductive function. As long ago as 1992, studies had addressed a possible action for NKB as a GnRH secretagogue; however, no evidence for this was found [20]. In more recent years, careful neuroanatomical studies had demonstrated NKB expression in key hypothalamic neurones in the infundibular or arcuate nucleus, which are highly responsive to sex steroids [21] and which co-express prodynorphin and the oestrogen receptor-α [21, 22]. Indirect evidence suggests that these neurones may also express KISS1, but this has yet to be directly demonstrated [23]. Furthermore, NK3Rs were shown to be expressed in GnRH nerve termini at the median eminence, where they are in close apposition to areas of NKB immunoreactivity [24].

However, although these studies place NKB and its receptor firmly at the scene of the crime, no smoking gun had been discovered directly linking NKB to normal function of the HPG axis prior to the recent human genetic studies: infusion of NKB into ovariectomised, oestrogen-primed rats failed to increase LH [25], and indeed may have suppressed it, in keeping with earlier studies [20]. Moreover, although any reproductive phenotype of *Tacr3* knockout mice has yet to be assessed in detail, existing data suggest that they do not exhibit impaired breeding efficiency [19 and Stock, pers. commun.]. This apparent major difference between the human and murine consequences of loss of NKB action must be borne in mind before overinterpreting neuroanatomical studies in rodents. The seemingly discordant reproductive consequences of loss of NKB action in mice and humans is also quite at odds with the situation seen for KISS1R, where murine genetic ablation of Kiss1r produces a faithful phenocopy of the human disease produced by KISS1R mutations [26]. This is particularly worthy of comment given the co-regulation of KISS1 and NKB by oestrogen, and their possible anatomical co-localisation in at least some of the key neurones that are believed to constitute the GnRH pulse generator [23], as well as the coupling of both KISS1 and NKB receptors to G_q-type G proteins and thence calcium flux.

Future Directions

These human and animal studies of NKB and its role in reproductive function are likely to be the beginning of concerted efforts to understand the biology at play in more detail. Progress is likely to be particularly rapid due to the investigational paradigm provided by studies of kisspeptin since 2003, and new reports are eagerly awaited in both humans and animals.

It will first be interesting to determine whether TACR3/TAC3 loss of function is indeed as prevalent in familial nIHH as suggested by the index human genetic studies. Identification of further mutations will permit more confident genotype-phenotype correlation, including assessment of differences between *TAC3* and *TACR3* loss of function, while studies of gonadotropin pulsatility, responses to exogenous GnRH, and ability to sustain a pregnancy of affected females will give further important human insights. It will also be intriguing to determine whether HH can be reversed in individuals with homozygous *TAC3* mutations by delivery of exogenous NKB, and further whether NKB can elicit a measurable gonadotropin response in healthy volunteers. Such studies would have to be undertaken with meticulous care, but the previous demonstration that NKB in pregnancy circulates at blood concentrations of up to around 120 pM [14] gives some confidence that careful systemic delivery of small doses of NKB is likely to be safe.

In order to tease out the precise molecular details of the action of NKB and its receptor in reproductive function, it will be essential to establish which available experimental organisms most reliably model human biology. Although mice are the most experimentally tractable species, the biology of their HPG axis differs markedly from that of humans and primates, and the preliminary evidence that *Tacr3–/–* mice have normal fertility [19 and Stock, pers. commun.] raises further concerns about the utility of murine studies – detailed reproductive assessment of *Tacr3* and *Tac2* null mice will be important in the first instance to clarify this. Primates provide the best model of human HPG function [27], but are much less widely available than mice. Nevertheless, preliminary evidence suggests that NKB may elicit a robust rise in LH in sheep [28], the best clue to date that NKB may indeed function as a GnRH secretagogue in at least some species contexts.

When an appropriate experimental model species has been validated for use, key questions will include whether there is a functional interaction between kisspeptin and NKB, and whether they function in series or in parallel. It will also be important to determine whether modulation of expression of NKB and its receptor may play a role as the proximal neural signal driving puberty, and whether agonists and antagonists can elicit potentially useful therapeutic effects.

Conclusions

In the last few years, careful studies in rodents have made a strong circumstantial case for a role for NKB and its endogenous receptor in the regulation of reproductive function. The very recent demonstration that human loss-of-function mutations in either NKB or its receptor produce profound HH further adds to this body of evidence by proving that intact NKB/NK3R function is absolutely required for normal human HPG action. However, this in vivo proof of the key reproductive role of NKB raises many new mechanistic questions, which future studies in humans and model organisms should seek to address in short order, aided by the recent paradigm provided by the past 6 years of study of kisspeptin and its receptor.

References

1 Semple RK, Topaloglu AK: The recent genetics of hypogonadotrophic hypogonadism – novel insights and new questions. Clin Endocrinol (Oxf) 2009, Epub ahead of print.
2 Seminara SB, Messager S, Chatzidaki EE, et al: The GPR54 gene as a regulator of puberty. N Engl J Med 2003;349:1614–1627.
3 de Roux N, Genin E, Carel JC, Matsuda F, Chaussain JL, Milgrom E: Hypogonadotropic hypogonadism due to loss of function of the KiSS1-derived peptide receptor GPR54. Proc Natl Acad Sci USA 2003;100: 10972–10976.
4 Crowley WF, Pitteloud N, Seminara SB: New genes controlling human reproduction and how you find them. Trans Am Clin Climatol Assoc 2008;119:29–38.
5 Topaloglu AK, Reimann F, Guclu M, Yalin AS, Kotan LD, Porter KM, Serin A, Mungan NO, Cook JR, Ozbek MN, Imamoglu S, Akalin NS, Yuksel B, O'Rahilly S, Semple RK: TAC3 and TACR3 mutations in familial hypogonadotropic hypogonadism reveal a key role for neurokinin B in the central control of reproduction. Nat Genet 2009;41:354–358.
6 Guran T, Tolhurst G, Bereket A, Rocha N, Porter KM, Turan S, Gribble FM, Kotan LD, Akcay T, Atay Z, Canan H, Serin A, O'Rahilly S, Reimann F, Semple RK, Topaloglu AK: A novel missense mutation in the first extracellular loop of the neurokinin B receptor causes hypogonadotropic hypogonadism. J Clin Endocrinol Metab 2009;94:3633–3639.
7 Prigge ST, Mains RE, Eipper BA, Amzel LM: New insights into copper monooxygenases and peptide amidation: structure, mechanism and function. Cell Mol Life Sci 2000;57:1236–1259.
8 Siuciak JA, McCarthy SA, Martin AN, Chapin DS, Stock J, Nadeau DM, Kantesaria S, Bryce-Pritt D, McLean S: Disruption of the neurokinin-3 receptor (NK3) in mice leads to cognitive deficits. Psychopharmacology (Berl) 2007;194:185–195.
9 Nordquist RE, Delenclos M, Ballard TM, Savignac H, Pauly-Evers M, Ozmen L, Spooren W: Cognitive performance in neurokinin 3 receptor knockout mice. Psychopharmacology (Berl) 2008;198:211–220.
10 Spooren W, Riemer C, Meltzer H: Opinion: NK3 receptor antagonists: the next generation of antipsychotics? Nat Rev Drug Discov 2005;4:967–975.
11 Panocka I, Massi M, Lapo I, Swiderski T, Kowalczyk M, Sadowski B: Antidepressant-type effect of the NK3 tachykinin receptor agonist aminosenktide in mouse lines differing in endogenous opioid system activity. Peptides 2001;22:1037–1042.
12 Ribeiro SJ, Teixeira RM, Calixto JB, De Lima TC: Tachykinin NK(3)receptor involvement in anxiety. Neuropeptides 1999;33:181–188.
13 Stoessl AJ, Dourish CT, Iversen SD: Pharmacological characterization of the behavioural syndrome induced by the NK-3 tachykinin agonist senktide in rodents: evidence for mediation by endogenous 5-HT. Brain Res 1990;517:111–1116.

14 Sakamoto R, Osada H, Iitsuka Y, Masuda K, Kaku K, Seki K, Sekiya S: Profile of neurokinin B concentrations in maternal and cord blood in normal pregnancy. Clin Endocrinol (Oxf) 2003;58:597–600.
15 Page NM, Woods RJ, Gardiner SM, Lomthaisong K, Gladwell RT, Butlin DJ, Manyonda IT, Lowry PJ: Excessive placental secretion of neurokinin B during the third trimester causes pre-eclampsia. Nature 2000;405:797–800.
16 Pennefather JN, Lecci A, Candenas ML, Patak E, Pinto FM, Maggi CA: Tachykinins and tachykinin receptors: a growing family. Life Sci 2004;74:1445–1463.
17 Pinto FM, Almeida TA, Hernandez M, Devillier P, Advenier C, Candenas ML: mRNA expression of tachykinins and tachykinin receptors in different human tissues. Eur J Pharmacol 2004;494:233–239.
18 Ding YQ, Lu BZ, Guan ZL, Wang DS, Xu JQ, Li JH: Neurokinin B receptor (NK3)-containing neurons in the paraventricular and supraoptic nuclei of the rat hypothalamus synthesize vasopressin and express Fos following intravenous injection of hypertonic saline. Neuroscience 1999;91:1077–1085.
19 Kung TT, Crawley Y, Jones H, Luo B, Gilchrest H, Greenfeder S, Anthes JC, Lira S, Wiekowski M, Cook DN, Hey JA, Egan RW, Chapman RW: Tachykinin NK3-receptor deficiency does not inhibit pulmonary eosinophilia in allergic mice. Pharmacol Res 2004;50:611–615.
20 Sahu A, Kalra SP: Effects of tachykinins on luteinizing hormone release in female rats: potent inhibitory action of neuropeptide K. Endocrinology 1992;130:1571–1577.
21 Goubillon ML, Forsdike RA, Robinson JE, Ciofi P, Caraty A, Herbison AE: Identification of neurokinin B-expressing neurons as a highly estrogen-receptive, sexually dimorphic cell group in the ovine arcuate nucleus. Endocrinology 2000;141:4218–4225.
22 Burke MC, Letts PA, Krajewski SJ, Rance NE: Coexpression of dynorphin and neurokinin B immunoreactivity in the rat hypothalamus: morphologic evidence of interrelated function within the arcuate nucleus. J Comp Neurol 2006;498:712–726.
23 Rance NE: Menopause and the human hypothalamus: evidence for the role of kisspeptin/neurokinin B neurons in the regulation of estrogen negative feedback. Peptides 2009;30:111–122.
24 Krajewski SJ, Anderson MJ, Iles-Shih L, Chen KJ, Urbanski HF, Rance NE: Morphologic evidence that neurokinin B modulates gonadotropin-releasing hormone secretion via neurokinin 3 receptors in the rat median eminence. J Comp Neurol 2005;489:372–386.
25 Sandoval-Guzman T, Rance NE: Central injection of senktide, an NK3 receptor agonist, or neuropeptide Y inhibits LH secretion and induces different patterns of Fos expression in the rat hypothalamus. Brain Res 2004;1026:307–312.
26 Chan YM, Broder-Fingert S, Seminara SB: Reproductive functions of kisspeptin and Gpr54 across the life cycle of mice and men. Peptides 2009;30:42–48.
27 Plant TM: Hypothalamic control of the pituitary-gonadal axis in higher primates: key advances over the last two decades. J Neuroendocrinol 2008;20:719–726.
28 McManus CJ, Valent M, Connors JM, Lehman MN, Goodman R: A neurokinin-B agonist stimulates LT secretion in follicular, but not luteal, phase ewes (abstract 760.8). Soc Neurosci Annu Meet, 2005, Washington.

Dr. Robert K. Semple
University of Cambridge Metabolic Research Laboratories
Institute of Metabolic Science, Addenbrooke's Hospital
Hills Road, Cambridge CB2 0QQ (UK)
Tel. +44 1223 769035, Fax +44 1223 330 598, E-Mail rks16@cam.ac.uk

Quinton R (ed): Kallmann Syndrome and Hypogonadotropic Hypogonadism.
Front Horm Res. Basel, Karger, 2010, vol 39, pp 142–153

Complex Genetics in Idiopathic Hypogonadotropic Hypogonadism

Nelly Pitteloud[a] · Sadia Durrani[a] · Taneli Raivio[b] · Gerasimos P. Sykiotis[a]

[a]Reproductive Endocrine Unit, Massachusetts General Hospital, Boston, Mass., USA; [b]Biomedicum Helsinki, Institute of Biomedicine and Physiology, University of Helsinki, Helsinki, Finland

Abstract

Idiopathic hypogonadotropic hypogonadism (IHH) is an important human disease model. Investigations of the genetics of IHH have facilitated insights into critical pathways regulating sexual maturation and fertility. IHH has been traditionally considered a monogenic disorder. This model holds that a single gene defect is responsible for the disease in each patient. In the case of IHH, 30% of cases are explained by mutations in one of eleven genes. In recent years, several lines of evidence have challenged the monogenic paradigm in IHH. First, disease-associated mutations display striking incomplete penetrance and variable expressivity within and across IHH families. Second, each locus is responsible for only a small percentage of cases. Third, more than one disease-associated mutation seems to be segregating in some families with IHH, and their combined or separate presence in individuals accounts for the variability in disease severity. Finally, IHH is not strictly a congenital and life-long disorder; occasionally it manifests itself during adulthood (adult-onset IHH); in other cases, the disease is not permanent, as evidenced by normal activity of the hypothalamic-pituitary-gonadal axis after discontinuation of treatment in adulthood (IHH reversal). Together, these observations suggest that IHH is not strictly a monogenic mendelian disease, as previously thought. Rather, it is emerging as a digenic, and potentially oligogenic disease, in which hormonal and/or environmental factors may critically influence genetic predisposition and clinical course. Future investigations of IHH should characterize the extent of the involvement of multiple genes in disease pathogenesis, and elucidate the contributions of epigenetic factors.

Investigations into the genetic basis of idiopathic hypogonadotropic hypogonadism (IHH) have been a rich vein for identifying genes and signaling pathways orchestrating the control of reproduction. In this manner, IHH has served as a unique model of neuroendocrine human disease from which insights into the genetic and molecular basis of reproductive physiology have been derived. For example, it is helping to elucidate the mechanisms regulating the timing of puberty, an intricate series of neuroendocrine events leading to attainment of adult height, maturation of secondary sex characteristics, and fertility. Although genetic factors are estimated to account for most of the normal variability in the timing of puberty, it remains a challenge to identify the specific underlying genes and regulatory networks [1]. The IHH paradigm has provided crucial insights directly from the human system that are shedding light on this great mystery of reproductive biology [2].

IHH is clinically defined as absent or incomplete puberty by the age of 18 years, resulting from low/normal or undetectable gonadotropin secretion in the setting of hypogonadal circulating sex hormone levels [3]. In nearly all cases, the primary reason for the dysfunction of the hypothalamic-pituitary-gonadal axis is deficiency in the production or action of gonadotropin-releasing hormone (GnRH), which leads to defective sexual maturation and infertility. Pulsatile GnRH therapy or gonadotropins can induce normal virilization and maturation of the gonads leading to fertility in >80% of cases [4]. The GnRH deficiency can be due to impaired fate specification from the olfactory placode, migration of the GnRH neurons to the hypothalamus during embryonic development, abnormal maturation of the GnRH network, decreased survival of GnRH neurons, or resistance to the action of GnRH at the level of the pituitary (see Chung and Tsai, this volume, pp. 37–50). IHH has been clinically divided into two major subtypes based on the presence or absence of a normal sense of smell: normosmic IHH (nIHH) or Kallmann syndrome with anosmia/hyposmia (KS). Moreover, sustained reversal of nIHH or KS can occur after discontinuation of therapy in adulthood (IHH reversal), or even develop after normal puberty (adult-onset IHH) [5–7]. IHH patients occasionally present with additional non-reproductive phenotypes, including midline craniofacial defects such as high-arched palate and cleft lip/palate, dental agenesis, bimanual synkinesis, renal agenesis, sensorineural hearing loss, and/or oculomotor abnormalities [8]. Thus, the constellation of additional non-reproductive phenotypes suggest that the genetic basis of IHH might also contribute to the pathogenesis of other associated diseases resulting in a multi-systemic syndrome.

IHH can present as either a sporadic or a familial disease [3]. The majority of IHH cases are sporadic (approximately 70%); in familial IHH, autosomal dominant, autosomal recessive, and X-linked recessive inheritance patterns have been described [9]. Traditionally, IHH has been considered a monogenic disorder, in which defects in one of a number of genes are responsible for the disease in affected individuals and families. The genes that have been implicated in the etiology of nIHH are *GNRHR* (encoding GnRH receptor, OMIM 138850), *GNRH1* (encoding pre-pro-GnRH, OMIM 152760), *GPR54* (G-protein-coupled receptor 54, OMIM 604161), *FGF8* (fibroblast growth factor 8, OMIM 600483), *FGFR1* (fibroblast growth factor receptor 1, OMIM 136350), *NELF* (nasal embryonic LHRH factor, OMIM 608137), *PROK2* (prokineticin 2, OMIM 607002), *PROKR2* (prokineticin receptor 2, OMIM 607212), *CHD7* (chromodomain helicase DNA-binding protein, OMIM 608892), *TAC3* (neurokinin B, OMIM 162330), and *TACR3* (neurokinin B receptor, OMIM 162330). Defects in four of the genes associated with nIHH, *FGF8*, *FGFR1*, *PROK2*, and *PROKR2* have also been shown to underlie KS; the gene implicated in X-linked recessive KS is *KAL1* (anosmin-1, OMIM 308700). Thus, it is now widely appreciated that IHH is characterized by significant genetic heterogeneity [10]. However, it is striking that mutation in each of these genes individually only accounts for a small proportion of IHH cases.

In addition to the genetic heterogeneity of IHH, genotype-phenotype relationships are variable. Specific mutant alleles show incomplete penetrance. Further, variable expressivity of both the reproductive and non-reproductive phenotypes within and across IHH families carrying the same gene defect have been reported. For example, certain gene defects have been found to underlie both nIHH and KS, even within the same family [11–15]. These observations strongly suggest that conventional monogenic inheritance cannot fully account for all the variability in the reproductive and non-reproductive phenotypes encountered in IHH patients. The genetic heterogeneity of IHH, the inconsistency of genotype-phenotype correlations, and the variability of the clinical course (including cases of adult-onset and reversal) strongly hint at the possibility that gene-gene and/or gene-environment interactions may underlie much of the pathogenic basis of IHH.

Next, we will review evidence demonstrating incomplete penetrance and variable expressivity of disease-associated mutations for many of the identified IHH genes. More detailed information on the discovery and function of each of these genes can be found in other chapters of the present volume.

Mutations Associated with Idiopathic Hypogonadotropic Hypogonadism Often Display Incomplete Penetrance and Variable Expressivity

KAL1

This was the first gene shown to cause the X-linked form of KS in about 10% of all male KS patients [16, 17]. Consistent with a critical role of KAL1/anosmin-1 in olfactory development and GnRH neuron migration [18], the reproductive phenotype of patient with *KAL1* mutations is often severe, with high frequency of cryptorchidism and microphallus, absent puberty, and infertility [19, 20]. *KAL1* mutations are highly penetrant, as in most cases men with mutations in the gene have KS. Interestingly, however, 3 brothers harboring the same *KAL1* deletion varied in terms of reproductive and olfactory phenotypes [21]. While 2 of the brothers failed to go through puberty and had anosmia, the 3rd one went through normal pubertal development and had only mild hyposmia. In addition, Sato et al. [22] described variable olfactory phenotypes in KS patients with *KAL1* mutations, and Ribeiro et al. [23] reported reversal of hypogonadism in a male proband with a premature stop codon in *KAL1*. The reason for the variable expressivity of the KS phenotype remains unclear; ostensibly, as yet unidentified modifier genes and/or environmental factors may compensate for the absence of KAL1 and thus prevent full expression of the KS phenotype. Further reports on variable expressivity of the non-reproductive phenotypes (renal agenesis, synkinesia, hearing loss) within family members carrying the same *KAL1* mutation have been published [8, 24, 25]. These cases have shown that even in a highly penetrant gene like *KAL1*, mutations do not always predict the clinical presentation (see also MacColl et al., this volume, pp. 62–77, and Choy and Kim, this volume, pp. 78–93).

GPR54

In 2003, two groups discovered GPR54 through linkage analysis as a critical gene involved in the onset of puberty [2, 26]. nIHH patients carrying either homozygous deletions or inactivating homozygous mutations in *GPR54* were reported. Very few nIHH cases have been described to date with *GPR54* mutations. One recent report is however consistent with variable expressivity. Five nIHH subjects from two unrelated kindreds carrying a homozygous L102P mutation exhibited variable reproductive phenotypes within and across kindreds [27] (see also Silveira et al., this volume, pp. 13–24, and Hameed and Dhillo, this volume, pp. 25–36).

FGFR1

In 2003, Dodé et al. [28] reported *FGFR1* as the first autosomal dominant gene underlying KS in about 10% of cases. Since then, numerous heterozygous *FGFR1* mutations underlying cases of KS [11, 12, 22, 29–31] and, more recently, also nIHH [13, 32] have been described. Frequent hallmarks of *FGFR1* mutations are marked reproductive and non-reproductive phenotypic variability both within and between families [12] carrying the same gene defect, and apparent incomplete penetrance [28]. For example, the R622X mutation in *FGFR1* has been reported in an nIHH kindred consistent with full penetrance and an autosomal dominant mode of inheritance [33]. The same mutation was reported by Dodé et al. [28] in a proband with KS and cleft palate and his apparently asymptomatic mother. Further, we have described the same mutation in a KS patient undergoing reversal, in his mother who had a history of delayed puberty, and his maternal grand-father with anosmia alone [11]. The ubiquitous expression of FGFR1 during development, including all along the GnRH neuron migratory path, may account for the variability in the reproductive and non-reproductive phenotypes associated with *FGFR1* mutations (see also Chung and Tsai, this volume, pp. 37–50, and Villanueva and de Roux, this volume, pp. 51–61).

FGF8

FGF8, a member of the FGF family, is a ligand for FGFR1; it has a wide range of biological functions, including a critical role as a morphogen in the developing brain [34, 35]. Recently, we have identified heterozygous and homozygous mutations in FGF8 underlying KS, nIHH, and also the adult-onset HH variant (AHH) [15]. Similarly to FGFR1, we reported variable expressivity within family members carrying the same gene defect. Further, we demonstrated an exquisite sensitivity of the GnRH neurons to decreased FGF8 signaling in vivo. Chung et al. [36] also showed that FGF8 signaling through FGFR1 is required for the early emergence of GnRH neurons from the embryonic olfactory placode (see also Chung and Tsai, this volume, pp. 37–50, and Villanueva and de Roux, this volume, pp. 51–61).

NELF
NELF (nasal epithelial LHRH factor) plays a key role in GnRH and olfactory neuron outgrowth [37, 38] and is co-localized with GnRH1 in human olfactory stem cells [39]. Only 2 cases of *NELF* mutations in IHH patients have been reported to date: a heterozygous missense mutation (T480A) whose biology remains unexplored [40], and an intronic deletion leading to defective mRNA expression [39].

PROK2 and PROKR2
Prokineticin-2 is a secreted protein which signals through the PROKR2 receptor and has functions in neuronal survival, circadian rhythms, and development of the olfactory and GnRH systems [29, 41]. In 2006, homozygous, compound heterozygous, and heterozygous mutations in PROK2 and PROKR2 were identified in patients with KS [42]. A homozygous loss-of-function in PROK2 has been reported in a kindred with both KS and nIHH, demonstrating variable expressivity of the disease. In this family, individuals carrying single defects in either PROK2 or PROKR2 were asymptomatic carriers [43]. In addition, several heterozygous mutations in PROK2 and PROKR2 have been reported in KS and nIHH with variable expressivity and incomplete penetrance, suggesting that these gene defects may not be sufficient to cause IHH (see also Sarfati et al., this volume, pp. 121–132).

CHD7
Mutations in *CHD7* underlie the severe congenital disorder CHARGE syndrome (coloboma, heart defects, choanal atresia, growth retardation, genitourinary abnormalities, ear abnormalities and deafness). CHD7 mutations occur in CHARGE patients who also exhibit the KS phenotype [44, 45]. Recently, *CHD7* mutations have been identified in subjects with nIHH [46]; however, a detailed phenotyping including an MRI of the auditory structures to exclude CHARGE syndrome was not reported. Further, the phenotypes of family members were not described, and thus it is not possible to comment on phenotypic variability (see also Aminzadeh et al., this volume, pp. 154–167).

TAC3 and TACR3
Very recently, autosomal recessive mutations in TACR3 were identified in four kindreds with nIHH, and an autosomal recessive mutation in TAC3 was found in a fifth kindred [47, 48]. The detailed phenotypes of subjects homozygous for either TAC3 or TACR3 mutations showed that all affected males had micropenis and cryptorchidism, suggesting a severe phenotype in these subjects. Further screening is warranted to assess the prevalence of mutations in these genes, and the degree of variable expressivity in IHH families.

GNRHR

This is the first gene discovered to cause nIHH inherited in an autosomal recessive form. Affected individuals are either homozygotes or compound heterozygotes for *GNRHR* mutations [49, 50], whereas family members carrying only one allelic defect appear asymptomatic. Phenotypic variability within and across family members carrying the same defect(s) in *GNRHR* have been reported. For example, de Roux et al. [49] described a patient and his sister that were compound heterozygotes for *GNRHR* mutations Q106R and R262Q; both exhibited partial nIHH, as evidenced by spontaneous testicular growth and active spermatogenesis in the brother and partial breast development in the sister. Notably, in a different kindred with affected family members carrying the same compound heterozygous mutations, 2 female patients exhibited absent puberty [51], a clearly more severe phenotype than that described by de Roux et al. [49]. Moreover, de Roux et al. [52] also described a family with affected members carrying the R262Q mutation in one *GNRHR* allele and two additional mutations (Q106R and A217R) in the other allele. Marked differences were observed in the reproductive phenotypes of the 3 patients who carried these mutations. Thus, variability in the reproductive phenotype has been described quite often in *GNRHR*. Interestingly, there is also a subset of nIHH patients who harbor heterozygous *GNRHR* mutations [53]. The significance of these mutations in nIHH pathogenesis remains unclear, but their presence indicates a more complex mode of inheritance than a single-gene disorder.

GNRH1

This was the first and most obvious nIHH candidate gene to be considered, but paradoxically the one to be most recently identified [54, 55]. The ability to rapidly and economically sequence entire genes in hundreds of unrelated probands was simply not available decades ago and, moreover, it was never anticipated that so many genes could each cause such a small percentage of the totality of nIHH cases. Three homozygote cases, 2 male and 1 female, from two (presumably) consanguineous kindreds of Near-Eastern origin, have been described so far, but data from other patient cohorts worldwide are not yet available. We simply do not know whether, for instance, compound heterozygotes for mutations in *GNRH1* and *GNRHR* exist and, if they do, whether they would exhibit the full phenotype of nIHH.

Limitations of Single-Gene Genotype-Phenotype Correlation Studies

The collective experience with genotype-phenotype correlations in IHH patients and their families suggests that a specific genotype at a single locus often cannot reliably predict the phenotype of the individual. This notion challenges traditional approaches to classification of the disease according to its phenotypic presentation and mode of inheritance. For example, since gene defects in several loci (*FGF8, FGFR1, PROK2, PROKR2*) can cause both KS and IHH, the distinction between KS and nIHH may simply represent variable expressivity of anosmia, a non-reproductive phenotype. Given that defects underlying IHH have been identified in less than 30% of IHH patients, it is conceivable that some, and perhaps even most, cases are caused by the interplay of several contributing genes. Next, we will discuss evidence in support of this model that has arisen from the identification of multiple mutations in several IHH patients.

Idiopathic Hypogonadotropic Hypogonadism Patients Can Harbor Pathogenic Mutations in More Than One Gene

In 2006, it was reported that a patient with sporadic KS who was heterozygous for the L173R mutation in *PROKR2* also carried a previously undescribed missense mutation in *KAL1* (S396L). Although the functional effects of the *KAL1* defect were not assessed, this mutation was not detected in 500 alleles from control individuals [42]. Shortly thereafter, the hypothesis of possible digenic inheritance in IHH was strengthened by the description of two additional kindreds [39]. In one kindred, a patient with KS carried heterozygous loss-of-function mutations in both *FGFR1* and *NELF*; in the other one, nIHH patients carried heterozygous mutations in *FGFR1* and compound heterozygous mutations in *GNRHR*. The discovery that these patients had defects in two genes rather than one helped explain the apparent lack of segregation of either gene with the disease in their respective families, and suggested that defects in different genes could 'co-operate' to produce a more severe phenotype than single-gene hits. Later, Falardeau et al. [15] reported 2 additional patients with nIHH carrying both an *FGFR1* mutation and an *FGF8* mutation. Since then, additional cases of digenicity have been reported, involving mutations in *PROKR2* with mutations in *PROK2* [56], *KAL1* [57, 58], *FGFR1*, *GPR54* and *GNRHR* [58]. More recently, Raivio et al. [manuscript under review] identified a truly multigenic IHH patient who carries compound heterozygous mutations in *GNRHR* and a heterozygous mutation in *FGFR1* as well as heterozygous *FGFR1* and *PROKR2* mutations.

The hitherto known cases of digenic defects in IHH patients are summarized in table 1. The involvement of multiple genes is a novel concept in IHH, and therefore its extent (percentage of patients with defects in more than one gene) and its degree (number of affected genes and alleles in each patient) remain to be characterized. This will require the comprehensive sequence analysis of all known IHH genes in large patient cohorts. If it turns out that defects in two or more genes are encountered with significant frequency, IHH may emerge as one of several human disorders which were originally considered monogenic, only to be later reclassified as oligogenic, i.e. caused by combinations of multiple gene defects. An early example of such model is retinitis pigmentosa, where mutations in both the *peripherin/RDS* and *ROM1* loci can synergize in disease pathophysiology [59]. There are now numerous further examples of oligogenicity in human disease, including such diverse disorders as Hirschsprung's [60], Bardet-Biedl syndrome [61], and nephronophthisis [62].

Table 1. IHH with mutations in more than one gene

Year of publication	Reference	IHH genes with mutations	Diagnosis
2006	[42]	*PROKR2 + KAL1*	KS
2007	[39]	*FGFR1 + NELF*	KS
2007	[39]	*FGFR1 + GNRHR*	nIHH
2008	[15]	*FGF8 + FGFR1*	nIHH
2008	[15]	*FGF8 + FGFR1*	nIHH
2008	[56]	*PROK2 + PROKR2*	KS
2009, 2010	[57, 58]	*PROKR2 + KAL1*	KS
2010	[58]	*PROKR2 + FGFR1*	KS
2010	[58]	*PROKR2 + GNRHR*	KS
2010	[59]	*PROKR2 + GPR54*	KS
	unpubl. data from our group	*FGFR1 + GNRHR FGFR1 + PROKR2*	nIHH nIHH

Cases of Adult-Onset and Reversal Imply Epigenetic Components in Idiopathic Hypogonadotropic Hypogonadism Pathophysiology

Although IHH is thought to be primarily a congenital genetic condition, it has been well established that individuals who have undergone normal puberty and sexual maturation can develop isolated GnRH deficiency in adult life (adult-onset IHH) [7]. More recently, the converse phenomenon has also been observed: hypogonadism can reverse late in adult life in about 10% of male patients with IHH [5]. The mechanisms underlying the reversal are unclear, but prior treatment with androgen/hCG was the common denominator in all the patients who reversed, and might be a critical requirement. Strikingly, both AHH and HH reversal can also occur in subjects carrying a known gene defect, e.g. an *FGF8* mutation in AHH [15], and an *FGFR1* mutation in IHH reversal [5]. Taken together, these observations suggest that, at least in some cases, in addition to its genetic basis, the pathogenesis of IHH may have non-genetic components. These currently unknown determinants can either predispose to or protect from disease manifestation, and appear to be able to alter the course of the disease even in the presence of pathogenic genetic defects. Elucidation of the nature of the underlying hormonal and/or environmental factors and of the epigenetic mechanisms by which they exert their influences on GnRH biology would represent a major breakthrough.

Conclusions

As genes underlying IHH continue to be identified, it is becoming more evident that the genetics of the disease are not strictly mendelian, and may involve mutations in more than one gene, as well as interactions between genes, environmental and/or hormonal factors. In single-gene mendelian disorders, the inheritance pattern of a specific allelic defect in a kindred corresponds well to the inheritance pattern of the disease phenotype (e.g. autosomal dominant, or X-linked recessive). In future investigations into the genetics of IHH, it would be helpful to distinguish between these two concepts, because this linear genotype-phenotype correspondence does not hold true in digenic and oligogenic situations.

Although a more complex genetic model for IHH may be currently challenging to conceptualize and demonstrate, upcoming sequencing technologies and international consortia of IHH patients should in the near future facilitate its comprehensive investigation. This emerging genetic model also has significant clinical advantages. For example, it could eventually explain not only the genetic heterogeneity but also the broad clinical spectrum of GnRH deficiency, which ranges from delayed puberty to severe IHH as well as the broad spectrum of non-reproductive phenotypes associated with IHH. It may also better facilitate genetic counseling, which is currently hampered by the fact that identification of a single gene defect in an IHH patient does not by itself reliably predict the phenotype in other family members. Thus, adopting an operational framework in IHH genetics that goes beyond the single-gene disorder paradigm will be beneficial in terms of both more accurately modeling the genetics of the disease and more confidently counseling patients and their families.

References

1 Parent AS, Teilmann G, Juul A, Skakkebaek NE, Toppari J, Bourguignon JP: The timing of normal puberty and the age limits of sexual precocity: variations around the world, secular trends, and changes after migration. Endocr Rev 2003;24:668–693.

2 Seminara SB, Messager S, Chatzidaki EE, et al: The GPR54 gene as a regulator of puberty. N Engl J Med 2003;349:1614–1627.

3 Seminara SB, Hayes FJ, Crowley WF Jr: Gonadotropin-releasing hormone deficiency in the human (idiopathic hypogonadotropic hypogonadism and Kallmann's syndrome): pathophysiological and genetic considerations. Endocr Rev 1998;19: 521–539.

4 Pitteloud N, Hayes FJ, Dwyer AA, Boepple PA, Lee H, Crowley WF Jr: Predictors of outcome of long-term GnRH therapy in men with idiopathic hypogonadotropic hypogonadism. J Clin Endocrinol Metab 2002;87:4128–4136.

5 Raivio T, Falardeau J, Dwyer AA, Quinton R, Hayes FJ, Hughes VA, Cole LW, Pearce SH, Lee H, Boepple P, Crowley WF Jr, Pitteloud N: Reversal of idiopathic hypogonadotropic hypogonadism. N Engl J Med 2007;357:863–873.

6 Quinton R, Cheow HK, Tymms DJ, Bouloux PM, Wu FC, Jacobs HS: Kallmann's syndrome: is it always for life? Clin Endocrinol (Oxf) 1999;50:481–485.

7 Nachtigall LB, Boepple PA, Pralong FP, Crowley WF, Jr: Adult-onset idiopathic hypogonadotropic hypogonadism – a treatable form of male infertility. N Engl J Med 1997;336:410–415.

8 Quinton R, Duke VM, Robertson A, Kirk JM, Matfin G, de Zoysa PA, Azcona C, MacColl GS, Jacobs HS, Conway GS, Besser GM, Stanhope RG, Bouloux PM: Idiopathic gonadotrophin deficiency: genetic questions addressed through phenotypic characterization. Clin Endocrinol (Oxf) 2001;55: 163–174.

9 Waldstreicher J, Seminara SB, Jameson JL, Geyer A, Nachtigall LB, Boepple PA, Holmes LB, Crowley WF Jr: The genetic and clinical heterogeneity of gonadotropin-releasing hormone deficiency in the human. J Clin Endocrinol Metab 1996;81:4388–4395.
10 Hardelin JP, Dodé C: The complex genetics of Kallmann syndrome: KAL1, FGFR1, FGF8, PROKR2, PROK2, et al. Sex Dev 2008;2:181–193.
11 Pitteloud N, Acierno JS Jr, Meysing AU, Dwyer AA, Hayes FJ, Crowley WF Jr: Reversible Kallmann syndrome, delayed puberty, and isolated anosmia occurring in a single family with a mutation in the fibroblast growth factor receptor 1 gene. J Clin Endocrinol Metab 2005;90:1317–1322.
12 Pitteloud N, Meysing A, Quinton R, Acierno JS Jr, Dwyer AA, Plummer L, Fliers E, Boepple P, Hayes F, Seminara S, Hughes VA, Ma J, Bouloux P, Mohammadi M, Crowley WF Jr: Mutations in fibroblast growth factor receptor 1 cause Kallmann syndrome with a wide spectrum of reproductive phenotypes. Mol Cell Endocrinol 2006;254–255:60–69.
13 Pitteloud N, Acierno JS Jr, Meysing A, Eliseenkova AV, Ma J, Ibrahimi OA, Metzger DL, Hayes FJ, Dwyer AA, Hughes VA, Yialamas M, Hall JE, Grant E, Mohammadi M, Crowley WF Jr: Mutations in fibroblast growth factor receptor 1 cause both Kallmann syndrome and normosmic idiopathic hypogonadotropic hypogonadism. Proc Natl Acad Sci USA 2006;103:6281–6286.
14 Pitteloud N, Zhang C, Pignatelli D, Li JD, Raivio T, Cole LW, Plummer L, Jacobson-Dickman EE, Mellon PL, Zhou QY, Crowley WF Jr: Loss-of-function mutation in the prokineticin 2 gene causes Kallmann syndrome and normosmic idiopathic hypogonadotropic hypogonadism. Proc Natl Acad Sci USA 2007;104:17447–17452.
15 Falardeau J, Chung WC, Beenken A, et al: Decreased FGF8 signaling causes deficiency of gonadotropin-releasing hormone in humans and mice. J Clin Invest 2008;118:2822–2831.
16 Hardelin JP, Levilliers J, del Castillo I, Cohen-Salmon M, Legouis R, Blanchard S, Compain S, Bouloux PM, Kirk JM, Moraine C, Chaussain JL, Weissenbach J, Petit C: X chromosome-linked Kallmann syndrome: stop mutations validate the candidate gene. Proc Natl Acad Sci USA 1992;89:8190–8194.
17 Bick DP, Schorderet DF, Price PA, Campbell L, Huff RW, Shapiro LJ, Moore CM: Prenatal diagnosis and investigation of a fetus with chondrodysplasia punctata, ichthyosis, and Kallmann syndrome due to an Xp deletion. Prenat Diagn 1992;12:19–29.
18 Cariboni A, Pimpinelli F, Colamarino S, Zaninetti R, Piccolella M, Rumio C, Piva F, Rugarli EI, Maggi R: The product of X-linked Kallmann's syndrome gene (KAL1) affects the migratory activity of gonadotropin-releasing hormone (GnRH)-producing neurons. Hum Mol Genet 2004;13:2781–2791.
19 Salenave S, Chanson P, Bry H, Pugeat M, Cabrol S, Carel JC, Murat A, Lecomte P, Brailly S, Hardelin JP, Dodé C, Young J: Kallmann's syndrome: a comparison of the reproductive phenotypes in men carrying KAL1 and FGFR1/KAL2 mutations. J Clin Endocrinol Metab 2008;93:758–763.
20 Pitteloud N, Hayes FJ, Boepple PA, DeCruz S, Seminara SB, MacLaughlin DT, Crowley WF Jr: The role of prior pubertal development, biochemical markers of testicular maturation, and genetics in elucidating the phenotypic heterogeneity of idiopathic hypogonadotropic hypogonadism. J Clin Endocrinol Metab 2002;87:152–60.
21 Parenti G, Rizzolo MG, Ghezzi M, Di Maio S, Sperandeo MP, Incerti B, Franco B, Ballabio A, Andria G: Variable penetrance of hypogonadism in a sibship with Kallmann syndrome due to a deletion of the KAL gene. Am J Med Genet 1995;57:476–478.
22 Sato N, Katsumata N, Kagami M, et al: Clinical assessment and mutation analysis of Kallmann syndrome 1 (KAL1) and fibroblast growth factor receptor 1 (FGFR1, or KAL2) in five families and 18 sporadic patients. J Clin Endocrinol Metab 2004;89:1079–1088.
23 Ribeiro RS, Vieira TC, Abucham J: Reversible Kallmann syndrome: report of the first case with a KAL1 mutation and literature review. Eur J Endocrinol 2007;156:285–290.
24 Matsuo T, Okamoto S, Izumi Y, Hosokawa A, Takegawa T, Fukui H, Tun Z, Honda K, Matoba R, Tatsumi K, Amino N: A novel mutation of the KAL1 gene in monozygotic twins with Kallmann syndrome. Eur J Endocrinol 2000;143:783–787.
25 Oliveira LM, Seminara SB, Beranova M, Hayes FJ, Valkenburgh SB, Schipani E, Costa EM, Latronico AC, Crowley WF Jr, Vallejo M: The importance of autosomal genes in Kallmann syndrome: genotype-phenotype correlations and neuroendocrine characteristics. J Clin Endocrinol Metab 2001;86:1532–1538.
26 de Roux N, Genin E, Carel JC, Matsuda F, Chaussain JL, Milgrom E: Hypogonadotropic hypogonadism due to loss of function of the KiSS1-derived peptide receptor GPR54. Proc Natl Acad Sci USA 2003;100:10972–10976.
27 Tenenbaum-Rakover Y, Commenges-Ducos M, Iovane A, Aumas C, Admoni O, de Roux N: Neuroendocrine phenotype analysis in five patients with isolated hypogonadotropic hypogonadism due to a L102P inactivating mutation of GPR54. J Clin Endocrinol Metab 2007;92:1137–1144.

28 Dodé C, Levilliers J, Dupont JM, et al: Loss-of-function mutations in FGFR1 cause autosomal dominant Kallmann syndrome. Nat Genet 2003;33: 463–465.

29 Albuisson J, Pêcheux C, Carel JC, Lacombe D, Leheup B, Lapuzina P, Bouchard P, Legius E, Matthijs G, Wasniewska M, Delpech M, Young J, Hardelin JP, Dodé C: Kallmann syndrome: 14 novel mutations in KAL1 and FGFR1 (KAL2). Hum Mutat 2005;25:98–99.

30 Sato N, Hasegawa T, Hori N, Fukami M, Yoshimura Y, Ogata T: Gonadotrophin therapy in Kallmann syndrome caused by heterozygous mutations of the gene for fibroblast growth factor receptor 1: report of three families: case report. Hum Reprod 2005; 20:2173–2178.

31 Sato N, Ohyama K, Fukami M, Okada M, Ogata T: Kallmann syndrome: somatic and germline mutations of the fibroblast growth factor receptor 1 gene in a mother and the son. J Clin Endocrinol Metab 2006;91:1415–418.

32 Xu N, Qin Y, Reindollar RH, Tho SP, McDonough PG, Layman LC: A mutation in the fibroblast growth factor receptor 1 gene causes fully penetrant normosmic isolated hypogonadotropic hypogonadism. J Clin Endocrinol Metab 2007;92:1155–1158.

33 Trarbach EB, Costa EM, Versiani B, de Castro M, Baptista MT, Garmes HM, de Mendonca BB, Latronico AC: Novel fibroblast growth factor receptor 1 mutations in patients with congenital hypogonadotropic hypogonadism with and without anosmia. J Clin Endocrinol Metab 2006;91:4006–4012.

34 Ornitz DM, Itoh N: Fibroblast growth factors. Genome Biol 2001;2:reviews3005.1–3005.12.

35 Mason I: Initiation to end point: the multiple roles of fibroblast growth factors in neural development. Nat Rev Neurosci 2007;8:583–596.

36 Chung WC, Moyle SS, Tsai PS: Fibroblast growth factor 8 signaling through fibroblast growth factor receptor 1 is required for the emergence of gonadotropin-releasing hormone neurons. Endocrinology 2008;149:4997–5003.

37 Kramer PR, Wray S: Novel gene expressed in nasal region influences outgrowth of olfactory axons and migration of luteinizing hormone-releasing hormone (LHRH) neurons. Genes Dev 2000;14:1824–1834.

38 Wray S: Molecular mechanisms for migration of placodally derived GnRH neurons. Chem Senses 2002;27:569–572.

39 Pitteloud N, Quinton R, Pearce SH, et al: Digenic mutations account for variable phenotypes in idiopathic hypogonadotropic hypogonadism. J Clin Invest 2007;117:457–463.

40 Miura K, Acierno JS Jr, Seminara SB: Characterization of the human nasal embryonic LHRH factor gene, NELF, and mutation screening among 65 patients with idiopathic hypogonadotropic hypogonadism (IHH). J Hum Genet 2004;49: 265–268.

41 Maldonado-Perez D, Evans J, Denison F, Millar RP, Jabbour HN: Potential roles of the prokineticins in reproduction. Trends Endocrinol Metab 2007;18:66–72.

42 Dodé C, Teixeira L, Levilliers J, et al: Kallmann syndrome: mutations in the genes encoding prokineticin-2 and prokineticin receptor-2. PLoS Genet 2006;2:e175.

43 Pitteloud N, Zhang C, Pignatelli D, Li JD, Raivio T, Cole LW, Plummer L, Jacobson-Dickman EE, Mellon PL, Zhou QY, Crowley WF Jr: Loss-of-function mutation in the prokineticin 2 gene causes Kallmann syndrome and normosmic idiopathic hypogonadotropic hypogonadism. Proc Natl Acad Sci USA 2007;104:17447–17452.

44 Jongmans MC, van Ravenswaaij-Arts CM, Pitteloud N, Ogata T, Sato N, Claahsen-van der Grinten HL, van der Donk K, Seminara S, Bergman JE, Brunner HG, Crowley WF Jr, Hoefsloot LH: CHD7 mutations in patients initially diagnosed with Kallmann syndrome – the clinical overlap with CHARGE syndrome. Clin Genet 2009;75:65–71.

45 Ogata T, Fujiwara I, Ogawa E, Sato N, Udaka T, Kosaki K: Kallmann syndrome phenotype in a female patient with CHARGE syndrome and CHD7 mutation. Endocr J 2006;53:741–743.

46 Kim HG, Kurth I, Lan F, Meliciani I, Wenzel W, Eom SH, Kang GB, Rosenberger G, Tekin M, Ozata M, Bick DP, Sherins RJ, Walker SL, Shi Y, Gusella JF, Layman LC: Mutations in CHD7, encoding a chromatin-remodeling protein, cause idiopathic hypogonadotropic hypogonadism and Kallmann syndrome. Am J Hum Genet 2008;83:511–519.

47 Topaloglu AK, Reimann F, Guclu M, Yalin AS, Kotan LD, Porter KM, Serin A, Mungan NO, Cook JR, Ozbek MN, Imamoglu S, Akalin NS, Yuksel B, O'Rahilly S, Semple RK: TAC3 and TACR3 mutations in familial hypogonadotropic hypogonadism reveal a key role for Neurokinin B in the central control of reproduction. Nat Genet 2009;41:354–358.

48 Guran T, Tolhurst G, Bereket A, Rocha N, Porter KM, Turan S, Gribble FM, Kotan LD, Akcay T, Atay Z, Canan H, Serin A, O'Rahilly S, Reimann F, Semple RK, Topaloglu AK: A novel missense mutation in the first extracellular loop of the neurokinin B receptor causes hypogonadotropic hypogonadism. J Clin Endocrinol Metab 2009;94:3633–3639.

49 de Roux N, Young J, Misrahi M, Genet R, Chanson P, Schaison G, Milgrom E: A family with hypogonadotropic hypogonadism and mutations in the gonadotropin-releasing hormone receptor. N Engl J Med 1997;337:1597–1602.

50 Layman LC, Cohen DP, Jin M, Xie J, Li Z, Reindollar RH, Bolbolan S, Bick DP, Sherins RJ, Duck LW, Musgrove LC, Sellers JC, Neill JD: Mutations in the gonadotropin-releasing hormone receptor gene cause hypogonadotropic hypogonadism. Nat Genet 1998;18:14–15.
51 Seminara SB, Beranova M, Oliveira LM, Martin KA, Crowley WF Jr, Hall JE: Successful use of pulsatile gonadotropin-releasing hormone (GnRH) for ovulation induction and pregnancy in a patient with GnRH receptor mutations. J Clin Endocrinol Metab 2000;85:556–562.
52 de Roux N, Young J, Brailly-Tabard S, Misrahi M, Milgrom E, Chaison G: The same molecular defects of the gonadotropin-releasing hormone gene determine a variable degree of hypogonadism in affected kindreds. J Clin Endocrinol Metab 1999;84:567–572.
53 Cerrato F, Shagoury J, Kralickova M, Dwyer AA, Falardeau J, Ozata M, Van Vliet G, Bouloux PM, Hall JE, Hayes FJ, Pitteloud N, Martin KA, Welt C, Seminara SB: Coding sequence analysis of GNRHR and GPR54 in patients with congenital and adult-onset forms of hypogonadotropic hypogonadism. Eur J Endocrinol 2006;155(suppl 1):S3–S10.
54 Bouligand J, Ghervan C, Tello J, Brailly-Tabard S, Salenave S, Chanson P, Lombès M, Millar RM, Guiochon-Mantel A, Young J: Familial isolated hypogonadotropic hypogonadism caused by a mutation in the gonadotropin-releasing hormone gene 1. N Engl J Med 2009;360:2742–2748.
55 Chan YM, de Guillebon A, Lang-Muritano M, Plummer L, Cerrato F, Tsiaras S, Gaspert A, Lavoie HB, Wu CH, Crowley WF Jr, Amory JK, Pitteloud N, Seminara SB: GNRH1 mutations in patients with idiopathic hypogonadotropic hypogonadism Proc Natl Acad Sci USA 2009;106:11703–11708.
56 Cole LW, Sidis Y, Zhang C, Quinton R, Plummer L, Pignatelli D, Hughes VA, Dwyer AA, Raivio T, Hayes FJ, Seminara SB, Huot C, Alos N, Speiser P, Takeshita A, Van Vliet G, Pearce SH, Crowley WF Jr, Zhou QY, Pitteloud N: Mutations in prokineticin 2 (PROK2) and PROK2 receptor (PROKR2) in human gonadotropin-releasing hormone deficiency: molecular genetics and clinical spectrum. J Clin Endocrinol Metab 2008;93:3551–3559.
57 Canto P, Munguía P, Söderlund D, Castro JJ, Méndez JP: Genetic analysis in patients with Kallmann syndrome: coexistence of mutations in prokineticin receptor 2 and KAL1. J Androl 2009;30:41–45.
58 Sarfati J, Guichon-Mantel A, Rondard P, et al: A comparative phenotypic study of Kallmann syndrome patients carrying monoallelic and biallelic mutations in the prokineticin 2 (PROK2) or prokineticin receptor 2 (PROKR2) genes. J Clin Endocrinol Metab 2010;[epub ahead of print].
59 Dryja TP, Hahn LB, Kajiwara K, Berson EL: Dominant and digenic mutations in the peripherin/RDS and ROM1 genes in retinitis pigmentosa. Invest Ophthalmol Vis Sci 1997;38:1972–1982.
60 Parisi MA, Kapur RP: Genetics of Hirschsprung disease. Curr Opin Pediatr 2000;12:610–617.
61 Katsanis N: The oligogenic properties of Bardet-Biedl syndrome. Hum Mol Genet 2004;13:R65–R71.
62 Hoefele J, Wolf MT, O'Toole JF, Otto EA, Schultheiss U, Deschenes G, Attanasio M, Utsch B, Antignac C, Hildebrandt F: Evidence of oligogenic inheritance in nephronophthisis. J Am Soc Nephrol 2007;18: 2789–2795.

Nelly Pitteloud, MD
Reproductive Endocrine Unit, Massachusetts General Hospital
55 Fruit Street
Boston, MA 02114 (USA)
Tel. +1 617 7263038, Fax +1 617 7265357, E-Mail npitteloud@partners.org

Quinton R (ed): Kallmann Syndrome and Hypogonadotropic Hypogonadism.
Front Horm Res. Basel, Karger, 2010, vol 39, pp 154–167

Rarer Syndromes Characterized by Hypogonadotropic Hypogonadism

Majid Aminzadeh[a] · Hyung-Goo Kim[b] ·
Lawrence C. Layman[b] · Timothy D. Cheetham[c]

[a]Division of Endocrinology and Metabolism, Abuzar Children's Hospital, Jundishapur University of Medical Sciences, Ahvaz, Iran; [b]Infertility and Genetics Section, Department of Obstetrics and Gynecology, Developmental Neurobiology Program, Institute of Molecular Medicine and Genetics, Neuroscience Program, Medical College of Georgia, Augusta, Ga., USA; [c]Institute of Human Genetics, University of Newcastle-upon-Tyne, Newcastle-upon-Tyne, UK

Abstract

Hypogonadotropic hypogonadism (HH) secondary to hypothalamic gonadotropin-releasing hormone deficiency is a notable feature of a number of rare syndromes, where unlike idiopathic (isolated) HH, other endocrinopathies may also be apparent. The presence of a particular spectrum of clinical features in addition to HH may suggest a particular underlying diagnosis. Placing the diagnosis of HH into that context will then have important implications in terms of management and predicting long-term functional outcome. In some instances, establishing the genetic basis of a particular syndrome or disorder has advanced the understanding of normal hypothalamo-pituitary-gonadal function (e.g. LEP deficiency, DAX-1 and CHARGE syndrome) whilst in other disorders much has still to be learnt (e.g. Bardet-Biedl and Prader-Willi syndrome). In this chapter the above syndromes, where HH is a feature in most or all affected individuals, will be discussed. Recent advances in our understanding of the pathophysiology of the HH will be highlighted and management options presented. Longer term therapy with sex steroid replacement is becoming even more important if improvements in life expectancy are to be matched by improvements in quality of life.

Hypogonadotropic hypogonadism (HH) is not always an isolated phenomenon, and in this chapter we will focus on five syndromes where most individuals also have HH. Pediatric endocrinologists can expect to encounter at least four of these disorders on a regular basis during their professional careers, and so an awareness of the various manifestations and management of associated sex steroid deficiency is likely to be useful. Moreover, their experience can be remarkably useful to the adult endocrinologist managing rarer and atypical disease presentation in later life.

Prader-Willi Syndrome (OMIM 176270)

Introduction

Prader-Willi syndrome (PWS) is the most common syndromic cause of obesity. The disorder is almost always sporadic with males and females affected equally. The clinical picture is quite characteristic with reduced fetal movements in utero and reduced muscle tone and activity levels in infancy. Excessive sleepiness, feeding problems and poor weight gain in early life are followed by a compulsion to eat with excessive weight gain. Tantrums, stubbornness and mood swings are observed in later childhood and adolescence. The clinical manifestations of HH are usually apparent by this time. Adults have mild learning difficulties and are usually hyperphagic and overweight or obese. Survival beyond the sixth decade is unusual [1].

Genetics

PWS was the first genetic disorder attributed to genomic imprinting and reflects loss or abnormal expression of the paternal copy of genes in the region of chromosome 15q11.2 –q13. At least five genes subject to genomic imprinting lie in this region and are implicated in PWS. The maternal genes in this region are normally inactivated through DNA methylation (imprinting), and there are three principle pathogenic mechanisms giving rise to 'loss' of paternal genes. The first is deletion of the PWS region on chromosome 15 normally inherited from the father (70% of patients). The second mechanism is where both copies of chromosome 15 are inherited from mother with no paternal PWS region (uniparental disomy – 25% of patients). Thirdly, the PWS phenotype can reflect a defect of the normal imprinting mechanism (<5% of cases). Most of these defects are 'epimutations' and hence are not associated with an abnormal DNA sequence, though in a minority of cases a microdeletion affects the imprinting centre.

Hypogonadism

Cryptorchidism occurs in 90% of boys and is usually bilateral. There may be associated micropenis, whilst most females have labial and clitoral hypoplasia (75%). Premature adrenarche is common, perhaps because of increased adiposity. Boys progress into puberty spontaneously but tend to arrest in mid-puberty with low or low-normal testosterone levels. Girls progress into puberty spontaneously, although this is frequently delayed. Breast development can be complete, although the breast is typically small or flat. Periods in girls are absent or irregular.

Pathophysiology

Normal urethral closure and labioscrotal fusion suggest that testosterone production in utero is normal. Low inhibin and high FSH levels can be found in some patients, possibly reflecting an element of primary gonadal dysfunction, Sertoli and/or defective germ cell maturation [2]. Testicular biopsy demonstrates Sertoli cells with a dearth of germ cells. Rodent studies have shown that disruption of *Necdin*, an imprinted gene located in the PWS region results in a 30% reduction in gonadotropin-releasing hormone (GnRH) neurons in the hypothalamus [3, 4].

Although the clinical picture is in keeping with HH, unlike in patients with classical idiopathic (isolated) HH (IHH) gonadotropin production can often be promoted with central estrogen antagonists, such as clomiphene citrate, by aromatase inhibition, or even by selective serotonin reuptake inhibitors, such as citalopram. These agents may induce ovulation and even pregnancy in females, and spermatogenesis in males.

Management Including Sex Steroid Replacement

Localization of testes with the help of an experienced sonographist may be useful if the testes cannot be palpated. In a few instances, MRI may give additional information prior to exploratory laparoscopy. A single random testosterone, FSH, LH and antimullerian hormone (AMH) are occasionally helpful, but most people feel that surgical exploration is warranted regardless. Risk of cancer in cryptorchid testes increases after puberty and early orchidopexy is preferred. Although future fertility is not a major issue for most individuals, an increased risk of torsion and psychosocial and cosmetic considerations are reasons why surgical intervention is important. Microphallus (stretched penis less than 2–3 cm) can be treated by 2–4 doses of 25 mg depot testosterone intramuscularly spaced 4 weeks apart.

Although there is a relative dearth of objective information regarding the advantages and disadvantages of testosterone replacement, there are good reasons to consider replacement in adolescence. The impact on behavioral problems needs to be considered (potentially good and bad) as well positive effects on secondary sexual characteristics and the skeleton (see below). Replacement should be considered by around 13–14 years of age. 25, then 50 mg depot testosterone monthly, increased carefully up to 100 mg every 1–2 weeks over the course of 3–4 years is one approach. It may, however, be appropriate to use a sub-replacement dose in some circumstances. Testosterone gels have their advocates, but we have also found the tablets (testosterone undecanoate, 40–80 mg daily) useful during adolescence and beyond. HCG (500–1,500 IU twice weekly) has also been used to complete puberty, with the authors reporting beneficial effects on muscle mass with no deterioration during therapy. Testosterone levels on HCG after 2 years ranged from 7.1 to 16 nM [5].

In females, signs of hypogonadism such as absent breast development, oligomenorrhea, or amenorrhea (primary or secondary) may warrant intervention with oral or dermal estrogen preparations combined with progestin. Careful monitoring during replacement therapy is mandatory. Although a small number of cases of pregnancies have been reported in females, no males with PWS are known to have fathered children.

Some of the key factors that optimize bone accretion, such as growth hormone (GH), exercise and gonadal steroid production may all be impaired in PWS, thus predisposing patients to reduced bone accrual and accelerated bone loss. Monitoring bone density and the optimization of remediable factors such as the intake of calcium and vitamin D, and GH and gonadal steroid replacement is crucial. Therapy with bisphosphonates for osteoporosis may be considered in later life.

CHARGE Syndrome (OMIM 214800)

Introduction

In 1981, the term 'CHARGE *association*' was used to describe a pattern of birth defects in children with the initials highlighting cardinal components. The initial description was of children with coloboma, heart defects, atresia of the choanae, retardation of growth and development, genital anomaly and ear abnormalities [6] but more refined clinical criteria for diagnosis were developed and reported by Blake et al. [7] with later modifications suggested by Verloes [8]. These criteria are summarized in tables 1 and 2. Now that the pathogenetics of CHARGE have been clearly established and the pattern of multiple anomalies known to be pathogenetically related, the correct term is 'CHARGE *syndrome*'.

The prevalence of CHARGE is approximately 1 in 10,000, and more than 400 patients have now been reported. Most patients with CHARGE syndrome have HH. Other aspects of pituitary function including GH and ACTH production are usually normal, although cases of GHD as well as primary and secondary hypothyroidism have been described [9].

Genetics

Mutations in the chromodomain helicase DNA binding protein 7 gene *(CHD7)*, located on chromosome 8q12.1, can be identified in the majority of patients with CHARGE syndrome. Most cases of CHARGE syndrome are sporadic, but transmission from individuals with a mild phenotype has been reported. The *CHD7* gene encodes a protein that probably regulates gene activity by chromatin remodeling. Most of the 150 mutations identified so far in CHARGE syndrome lead to the production of an abnormally short, nonfunctional CHD7 protein. *CHD7* is expressed in many tissues including the semicircular canals, the forebrain, pituitary gland, olfactory bulbs and nerves, the nasal epithelia, the neural retina and the optic nerve sheath. It is likely that changes in gene expression during embryonic development cause the clinical features of CHARGE syndrome. Several explanations could explain the clinical picture in patients without mutations including genetic heterogeneity, intronic mutations in the *CHD7* gene, exon deletions or duplications (necessarily missed by sequencing) and 3′ or 5′ UTR mutations [9, 10].

Hypogonadism

Hypogonadism was known to be associated with CHARGE syndrome prior to the identification of *CHD7* [11]. However, it was only recently that heterozygous *CHD7* mutations were identified in patients with apparent normosmic HH (nIHH) and

Table 1. Clinical criteria with prevalence figures in brackets [7]

Major criteria	Minor criteria	Inclusion rule
Coloboma of the iris, retina, choroid or disc (75–90%) Microphthalmia	Hypoplastic genitalia – micropenis and cryptorchidism (80%) – hypoplastic labia (30–40%) HH (65–85%)	4 majors OR 3 majors + 3 minors
Choanal atresia (35–65%)	Developmental delay – delayed motor milestones – language delay – learning disability of varying degree	
Ear abnormalities (>95%) – external ear (lop or cup shaped) – middle ear (ossicular malformations; chronic serous otitis media) – inner ear (cochlear defects) – mixed deafness (60–90%)	Cardiovascular malformations – conotruncal defect, e.g. Fallot's tetralogy – AV canal defects – aortic valve or arch defects	
Cranial nerve dysfunction – unilateral or bilateral facial palsy – sensorineural deafness – swallowing problems	Growth deficiency – short stature – GH deficiency	
	Orofacial cleft (15–20%)	
	Tracheoesophageal fistula	
	Characteristic facies	

Kallmann syndrome (KS) [12, 13]. Initial studies supported a possible relationship between the KS phenotype and CHARGE syndrome. This evidence, detailed and referenced in Kim et al. [12], consisted of the following:

First, anosmia or hyposmia, sometimes with abnormal olfactory bulbs by MRI, has been identified in children with CHARGE syndrome. Second, most CHARGE boys studied had micropenis and/or cryptorchidism suggestive of IHH (although all were of prepubertal age). Third, none of 7 females >12 years old began puberty spontaneously, and hormonal data suggested the likelihood of IHH becoming evident as they got older. Finally, one female CHARGE patient with a *CHD7* mutation also had features of KS. These findings led Kim et al. [12] to hypothesize that some cases of nIHH and KS could represent milder allelic variants of CHARGE syndrome.

When 101 unrelated nIHH and KS patients without features of CHARGE syndrome were analyzed, heterozygous *CHD7* mutations, either splice or missense, were

Table 2. Clinical criteria with prevalence figures in brackets [8]

Major criteria	Minor criteria	Inclusion rule
Ocular coloboma	Rhombencephalic dysfunction Brainstem and cranial nerve III–XII anomalies, including sensorineural deafness	Typical CHARGE: 3 majors OR 2 majors + 2 minors
Choanal atresia	Hypothalamo-hypophyseal dysfunction (including GH and gonadotropin defects)	Partial CHARGE: 2 majors + 1 minor
Hypoplastic semicircular canals	Malformation of the ear Internal or external	Atypical CHARGE: 2 majors, but no minors OR 1 major + 2 minors
	Malformation of mediastinal organs Heart Tracheoesophageal	
	Learning disability	

identified in 6% of KS and 6% of nIHH patients [12]. In an additional 96 patients, exons 6–10 encoding the conserved chromodomains were sequenced, and one further mutation was identified. Some mutations affected chromodomains, which are thought to be critical for proper CHD7 function in chromatin remodeling and transcriptional regulation, while others affected conserved residues of the protein. Interestingly, CHARGE syndrome patients tended to have frameshift *CHD7* mutations [11], while nIHH/KS patients had less severe missense or splice mutations [12]. These findings indicated that both nIHH and KS are mild allelic variants of CHARGE syndrome caused by *CHD7* mutations. Therefore, IHH/KS patients should be examined carefully for phenotypic findings suggestive of CHARGE syndrome. Although the IHH/KS patients had sporadic inheritance, CHD7 mutations can cause autosomal dominant disease, so appropriate genetic counseling should be performed.

Pathophysiology

Gonadotropin deficiency is responsible for genital hypoplasia in male patients and for the lack of secondary sexual development in both sexes. The pattern of expression of *CHD7*, the observation that many patients with CHARGE syndrome have anosmia and/or an abnormal olfactory bulb on MRI, and the recent demonstration of *CHD7* mutations in KS patients, all suggest a pathophysiological link between KS and CHARGE. Anosmin has been found to regulate FGFR1 activity (see Chung and Tsai, this volume, pp. 37–50, Villanueva and de Roux, this volume, pp. 51–61, and MacColl et al., this volume, pp. 62–77), and it is possible that CHD7, in turn, controls the transcription of one or more genes encoding proteins involved in FGF signaling. Alternatively, FGF signaling through FGFR1 may control the activity of *CHD7* or its transcription in the olfactory bulb primordium. Thus, abnormal functioning of FGF pathways in both Kallmann and CHARGE syndromes may result in the failed embryonic migration of GnRH-synthesizing neurons along the olfactory nerve pathway resulting in HH.

Management Including Sex Steroid Replacement

Random and stimulated gonadotropin and testosterone measurements are typically low in teenage patients [10]. In male infants with cryptorchidism and micropenis, hCG treatment may assist testicular descent and penile development. If testicular descent is not achieved, then referral for orchidopexy is appropriate. Low-dose testosterone therapy in infancy will also help penile growth. Puberty should be induced at an appropriate age, initially with low-dose replacement, increased gradually as secondary sexual characteristics develop. More formal 'adult' replacement can then be commenced in later adolescence using one of the range of preparations available according to patient preference. Testosterone therapy should be continued indefinitely to maintain satisfactory bone and muscle mass, and to optimize well-being and cardiac function. Spermatogenesis induction is theoretically possible, though this might be compromised by earlier cryptorchidism.

In females, pubertal induction should begin with low-dose unopposed estrogen replacement, increased progressively until an 'adult' dose is achieved. Satisfactory breast development and/or break-through bleeding warrant the addition of a progestogen. There are a range of adult replacement estrogen/progesterone preparations available including the combined pill. The choice will clearly reflect the discussions between physician and patient. Administration of estrogen until the age of menopause is necessary to maintain bone density, and adequacy of replacement can be assessed by DEXA scanning. Ovulation induction may be achievable through standard protocols.

Congenital Adrenal Hypoplasia and DAX-1 (OMIM 300200)

Introduction

The terms adrenal hypoplasia congenita (AHC) or congenital adrenal hypoplasia refer to individuals with adrenal insufficiency who do not have an underlying steroidogenic defect such as 21 hydroxylase deficiency and who do not have autoimmune adrenal damage or infiltration. Congenital adrenal hypoplasia is usually due to deletions or mutations in the *DAX1* (*NR0B1*) gene on the X chromosome (dosage-sensitive sex reversal AHC critical region on the X chromosome, gene 1) [14, 15], and over 100 cases have been described. Adrenal insufficiency commonly presents in the neonatal period or in childhood. Aldosterone deficiency usually precedes cortisol deficiency, and so many patients present with salt wasting. Males may have cryptorchidism, micropenis and hypospadias. X-linked AHC can present in adult life with abnormal gonadal, rather than adrenal function, as the presenting problem.

Genetics

The *DAX1* gene is located at Xp21.3-Xp21.2. DAX-1 is an orphan nuclear receptor and does not have the typical zinc finger DNA-binding domain seen in other members of the nuclear receptor superfamily. It is expressed in the hypothalamus, hypophysis, adrenal cortex and gonads. The DAX-1 protein functions as a transcriptional repressor of a number of genes including steroidogenic factor-1. Missense, frameshift, nonsense mutations and deletions of the *DAX1* gene *(NROB)* are reported in AHC as well as contiguous gene defects involving neighboring genes such as glycerol kinase and Duchenne muscular dystrophy. Duplication of *DAX-1* results in partial or complete dosage-sensitive sex reversal syndrome in 46XY fetuses (by inhibition of both testosterone and AMH production). DAX-1 exists in a complex genetic network that makes it difficult to predict phenotype from genotype. The synergistic interaction of steroidogenic factor-1 and Wilms' tumor-1 proteins on AMH during male sexual development is antagonized by DAX-1. A skewed X-inactivation pattern can occasionally result in girls being affected [16].

Hypogonadism

Patients have primary gonadal failure in addition to gonadotropin deficiency. Microphallus and undescended testes can be seen in infancy, although several reports have described normal hypothalamic-gonadotroph-Leydig cell axis function in infancy [17]. All studies have reported absent, delayed or partial puberty in boys with low testosterone, low gonadotropins and a poor or absent response to GnRH stimulation (except in 2 cases). Thus, abnormalities in the hypothalamic-gonadotroph axis appear to evolve. Testicular volume in adults is pathologically small but may exceed 4 ml.

The presentation of patients with *DAX1* defects is heterogeneous, with adrenal failure first occurring in infancy, childhood or even in adult life [18]. Although gonadotropin deficiency may be partial, there is no meaningful spermatogenetic response to gonadotropin treatment. Hence, an element of primary testicular failure can be inferred, independent of any dysfunction arising from cryptorchidism. The clinical spectrum also includes 'simple' delayed puberty in females, IHH with intact adrenal function in females and isolated mineralocorticoid deficiency in males (unusual mutation in aminoterminus). Screening for *DAX1* mutations in IHH patient series (without adrenal failure) has not identified any cases to date. Gonadotropin-independent precocious puberty has been reported and may reflect chronic excessive ACTH stimulation of Leydig cells [19].

Pathophysiology

The ligand for DAX-1 is unknown, hence the term orphan nuclear receptor. *Dax-1* null mice do not demonstrate adrenal hypoplasia and have normal gonadotropins, but males are sterile (due to progressive impairment in spermatogenesis), whereas females have normal fertility. It is unclear how loss of gene function results in loss of hypothalamic and adrenal cortical development in humans. Azoospermia is present and does not respond to gonadotropin treatment, indicating a role for DAX-1 in spermatogenesis independent of gonadotropins. The product of *DAX1* appears to suppress expression of the *SF1*-regulated steroidogenic acute regulatory protein promoter. *DAX1* also appears to function as an 'anti-testis' gene by acting antagonistically to the sex-determining region on the Y chromosome. Some studies suggest an inverse correlation between *DAX1* expression and the pattern of steroid hormone production in human adrenocortical tumors.

Management

The major focus initially will involve the assessment and management of any impaired adrenal function. Management of microphallus and undescended testis should be considered in infancy. Patients will, of course, need stress doses of glucocorticoid at the time of orchidopexy. As in other causes of HH, the best choice for induction of puberty is testosterone replacement therapy. Because of the wide range of severity of HH in these patients (late onset, incomplete to complete deficiency), it is better to evaluate the axis around the normal age of pubertal onset then treat according to height, bone age and individual preference. Virtually all males have azoospermia unresponsive to gonadotropin treatment, with no reports of fertility in this disorder, though occasional cases of oligospermia have been reported. Testosterone replacement treatment should be continued life-long.

Leptin Deficiency (OMIM 164160) and Resistance (OMIM 601007)

Introduction

Leptin from the Greek word *leptos*, meaning thin, is an adipocyte-secreted 16-kDa protein that provides information to the central nervous system regarding peripheral energy stores. It is also involved in a range of other diverse physiological processes including hematopoiesis, immune function and reproduction. Leptin acts through the leptin receptor (LEPR), a single-transmembrane domain receptor of the cytokine receptor family that is found in many tissues in several alternatively spliced forms. Serum leptin levels in boys appear to peak just before puberty or in early Tanner stages, followed by a decrease to baseline levels as testosterone levels rise.

Girls display a steady rise in leptin levels throughout puberty with a relationship between the onset of menarche and serum leptin levels. Each increase of 1 ng/ml in serum leptin is associated with an earlier onset of menarche by 1 month. The linkage between body fat and the reproductive axis in girls may have evolved in mammals as a mechanism for ensuring that pregnancy will not occur unless there are adequate fat stores to sustain both the mother and the growing fetus. Leptin has a diurnal rhythm, with peak serum concentrations in early morning hours and a nadir in the afternoon. Similar circadian patterns have been noted in both lean and obese individuals (with obese patients having higher pulse amplitude).

Genetics
The human leptin (Ob) gene consists of 3 exons and 2 introns and spans about 18 kb. The longest isoform of the leptin receptor (Ob-Rb) is a member of the interleukin-6 receptor family of class I cytokine receptors, which contains box1/box2 Janus kinase (JAK), signal transducers and activators of transcription binding sites for intracellular signal transduction. The short form contains only box1 JAK binding sites for JAK and MAPK activation. It is highly expressed in a more widespread fashion in peripheral tissues, and may mediate leptin clearance or leptin transport through the blood-brain barrier.

Human leptin deficiency was first described in the context of a homozygous deletion of a guanine nucleotide in the leptin gene between nucleotides 393 and 398 which disrupted the reading frame of the leptin gene, leading to the introduction of 14 aberrant amino acids after gly132 in the leptin polypeptide, followed by a premature stop codon [20]. A child has also been described who was found to be homozygous for a guanine deletion in codon 133 of leptin (delta-G133). There are known to be at least 12 patients worldwide with leptin deficiency. Defects in the leptin receptor are rather more common and have been identified in 3% of severe early-onset obesity cases. Unlike leptin deficiency, there is no 'magic bullet' treatment option for affected individuals [21].

Hypogonadism
Patients with leptin deficiency are obese with gonadotropin deficiency and late or absent puberty. Patients with leptin receptor defects are hyperphagic with severe obesity and also have altered immune function as well as delayed puberty due to HH. Final height is reduced, presumably because of an absent growth spurt. Clinical features of LEPRs are less severe than those of subjects with LEPD. Subjects with LEPRs do not experience menses until later life but this probably reflects aromatization of androgen rather than normal gonadotropin production. However, gonadotropin production does occur in patients with leptin receptor defects, suggesting that activation of the hypothalamo-pituitary-gonadal (HPG) axis is possible in the absence of leptin activity. Impaired HPG axis activity in females is more prominent than in males. Women suffer anovulation/irregular menses and impaired lactation, but fertility can be seen in men.

Pathophysiology
GnRH pulses are suppressed by food restriction, high or low ambient temperature and excessive exercise. GnRH pulsatility returns when such challenges are addressed. Leptin receptors are localized in several regions of the brain involved in energy regulation and reproductive function. This includes the arcuate nucleus/median eminence, paraventricular nucleus, and ventromedial nucleus. Leptin appears to act on two populations of cells in the arcuate nucleus. It has an inhibitory effect on NPY (an orexigenic peptide)-producing cells and stimulates POMC (an anorectic

neuropeptide)-producing cells. NPY neurons are activated under conditions of negative energy balance, leading to an increase in NPY release from terminals in the paraventricular nucleus and preoptic area. Increased NPY release may then stimulate feeding behavior while inhibiting release of GnRH. Leptin accelerates GnRH pulsatility, but not pulse amplitude, in arcuate hypothalamic neurons in a dose-dependent manner, and it is also possible that leptin stimulates KiSS-1 expression and stimulation of GnRH release. However, current evidence indicates that leptin plays a permissive role rather than acting as the critical metabolic signal initiating puberty. Hence, it is not the sole regulator of GnRH secretion, but works in concert with other molecules (see Silveira et al., this volume, pp. 13–24, and Hameed and Dhillo, this volume, pp. 25–36). Leptin receptors (Ob-Rs) are also present in the granulosa, theca, and interstitial cells of the ovary, endometrium and Leydig cells. Leptin levels correlate with fat content and hence are not a reliable marker for an underlying leptin receptor defect.

Management

Recombinant leptin administration to patients with leptin deficiency leads to a dramatic reduction in body mass index (BMI) and addresses all other aspects of the phenotype including abnormal gonadotropin release [22]. Leptin replacement 0.01–0.04 mg/kg once daily for 18 months in leptin-deficient adults has a profound impact on body weight. Individuals become more active, sexually mature and assertive. Medium-term use of leptin in children is safe and accompanied by continuous weight loss albeit with refractory periods overcome by an increase in leptin dose. More than 98% of weight loss was represented by fat mass.

A steady and consistent reduction in fasting plasma insulin occurs as fat mass falls, accompanied by a gradual increase in gonadotropins, estradiol and pubertal development in a girl with bone age equal to 12.5 without pubertal signs (but not in younger cases). These effects were seen at a dose equivalent to 10% of normal serum concentration. In women with exercise- or anorexia-induced amenorrhea, leptin treatment increases pulse frequency and levels of LH, ovarian volume and estradiol levels [23]. If leptin is unavailable and in cases of leptin receptor abnormalities, classical approaches to obesity and IHH, such as sex steroid replacement, will need to be considered.

Prohormone Convertase 1/3 Deficiency (OMIM 162150)

A large number of biologically inactive prohormones and neuropeptides are cleaved enzymatically by prohormone convertases to generate biologically active peptides. Congenital deficiency of the neuroendocrine-specific enzyme prohormone convertase (PC1/3), located at 5q15–21, has been reported as an autosomal recessive condition in three kindreds worldwide, with probands being homozygotes or compound heterozygotes for mutations of *PC1/3*, resulting in either truncated, non-secreted or functionally impaired protein product, respectively. PC1/3 deficiency is characterized by neonatal-onset enteropathy, dysregulated glucose homeostasis causing reactive hypoglycemia, early-onset hyperphagic obesity and impaired prohormone processing. The latter is biochemically manifest by a moderate degree of central hypothyroidism, hypocortisolemia and hypoinsulinemia, with elevated ratios of proinsulin/insulin and of POMC/ACTH. In addition, HH becomes evident after normal age of pubertal onset [24–26].

Bardet-Biedl Syndrome (OMIM 209900)

Introduction

Bardet-Biedl syndrome (BBS) is a rare developmental and progressive degenerative disorder with the cardinal features of rod-cone retinal dystrophy, abdominal obesity, postaxial polydactyly, cognitive impairment, renal and cardiac anomalies, hypertension and diabetes. Although primarily an autosomal recessive disorder, it is clinically and genetically heterogeneous disorder with 12 *BBS* genes identified to date and evidence for two additional functionally-related loci, *MKS1* and CEP290, resulting in a broadly similar phenotype. Abnormalities of all these genes impact on cilia and basal body function, hence the term 'ciliopathy' [27, 28].

Genetics

BBS is associated with mutations in genes at various loci including: 11q13 (*BBS1*: 209901), 16q21 (*BBS2*: 606151), the ADP-ribosylation factor gene on 3p12-q13 (*BBS3* or *ARL6*: 608845), 15q22.3 (*BBS4*: 600374), 2q31 (*BBS5*: 603650), 20p12 (*BBS6* or *MKKS* 604896), 4q27 (*BBS7*: 607590), a tetratricopeptide repeat domain-containing gene on chromosome 14q32.11 (*BBS8*: 608132), 7p14 (*BBS9*: 607968), 12q (*BBS10*: 610148), 9q33.1 (*BBS11*: 602290), 4q27 (*BBS12*: 610683), 17q23 (*MKS1* or *BBS13*: 609883), 12q21.3 (*CEP290* or *BBS14*: 610142). In addition, the *CCDC28B* gene (610162) modifies the expression of BBS phenotypes in patients who have mutations in other genes. The vast genetic heterogeneity of BBS renders molecular genetic diagnosis problematic due to time and cost required to screen upwards of 204 coding exons [27, 28].

Hypogonadism

Most male patients have a small phallus with around 10% in one series having cryptorchidism. Many women have menstrual irregularities, with some having low estrogen levels. Both secondary and primary gonadal failure is reported. Structural genital abnormalities are reported including persistent urogenital sinus, uterine hypoplasia and vaginal atresia. Suboptimal GH responses on provocation testing have been reported (although these patients tend to be obese), and testosterone responses to HCG are also low. Hence, both primary and secondary hypogonadism may be features of BBS. It is unclear why some patients with BBS have primary hypogonadism, although this presumably reflects abnormal ciliary function [27]. Patients should be managed according to their clinical and biochemical phenotype with an assessment of the HPG axis at adolescence. Hormone replacement with testosterone (males) or estrogen (females) may be appropriate.

References

1 Eiholzer U, Lee PDK: Medical considerations in Prader-Willi syndrome; in Butler MG, Lee PDK, Whitman BY (eds): Management of Prader-Willi Syndrome, ed 3. New York, Springer, 2006, pp 97–152.

2 Eiholzer U, l'Allemand D, Rousson V, Schlumpf M, Gasser T, Girard J, Grüters A, Simoni M: Hypothalamic and gonadal components of hypogonadism in boys with Prader-Labhart-Willi syndrome. J Clin Endocrinol Metab 2006;91:892–898.

3 Muscatelli F, Abrous DN, Massacrier A, Boccaccio I, Le Moal M, Cau P, Cremer H: Disruption of the mouse Necdin gene results in hypothalamic and behavioural alterations reminiscent of the human Prader-Willi syndrome. Hum Mol Genet 2000;9: 3101–3110.

4 Miller NL, Wevrick R, Mellon PL: Necdin, a Prader-Willi candidate gene, regulated gonadotropin-releasing hormone neurons during development. Hum Mol Genet 2009;18:248–260.

5 Eiholzer U, Grieser J, Schlumpf M, L'Allemand D: Clinical effects of treatment for hypogonadism in male adolescents with Prader-Labhart-Willi syndrome. Horm Res 2007;68:178–184.

6 Sanlaville D, Verloes A: CHARGE syndrome: an update. Eur J Hum Genet 2007;15:389–399.

7 Blake KD, Davenport SLH, Hall BD, Hefner MA, Pagon RA, Williams MS, Lin AE, Graham JM: CHARGE association: an update and review for the primary pediatrician. Clin Pediatr 1998;37:59–173.

8 Verloes A: Updated diagnostic criteria for CHARGE syndrome: a proposal. Am J Med Genet 2005;133A: 306–308.

9 Asakura Y, Toyota Y, Muroya K, Kurosawa K, Fujita K, Aida N, Kawame H, Kosaki K, Adachi M: Endocrine and radiological studies in patients with molecularly confirmed CHARGE syndrome. J Clin Endocrinol Metab 2008;93:920–924.

10 Wheeler PG, Quigley CA, Sadeghi-Nejad A, Weaver DD: Hypogonadism and CHARGE association. Am J Med Genet 2000;94:228–231.

11 Vissers LE, van Ravenswaaij CM, Admiraal R, Hurst JA, de Vries BB, Janssen IM, van der Vliet WA, Huys EH, de Jong PJ, Hamel BC, Schoenmakers EF, Brunner HG, Veltman JA, van Kessel AG: Mutations in a new member of the chromodomain gene family cause CHARGE syndrome. Nat Genet 2004;36:955–957.

12 Kim HG, Kurth I, Lan F, Meliciani I, Wenzel W, Eom SH, Kang GB, Rosenberger G, Tekin M, Ozata M, Bick DP, Sherins RJ, Walker SL, Shi Y, Gusella JF, Layman LC: Mutations in CHD7, encoding a chromatin-remodeling protein, cause idiopathic hypogonadotropic hypogonadism and Kallmann syndrome. Am J Hum Genet 2008;83:511–519.

13 Jongmans MC, van Ravenswaaij-Arts CM, Pitteloud N, Ogata T, Sato N, Claahsen-van der Grinten HL, van der Donk K, Seminara S, Bergman JE, Brunner HG, Crowley WF Jr, Hoefsloot LH: CHD7 mutations in patients initially diagnosed with Kallmann syndrome – the clinical overlap with CHARGE syndrome. Clin Genet 2009;75:65–71.

14 Zanaria, E, Muscatelli F, Bardoni B, Strom TM, Guioli S, Guo W, Lalli E, Moser C, Walker AP, McCabe ER Meitinger T, Monaco AP, Sassone-Corsi P, Camerino G: An unusual member of the nuclear hormone receptor superfamily responsible for X-linked adrenal hypoplasia congenita. Nature 1994;372:635–641.

15 Muscatelli F, Strom TM, Walker AP, Zanaria E, Récan D, Meindl A, Bardoni B, Guioli S, Zehetner G, Rabl W, Schwarz HP, Kaplan JC, Camerino G, Meitinger T, Monaco AP: Mutations in the DAX1 gene give rise to both X-linked adrenal hypoplasia congenita and hypogonadotropic hypogonadism. Nature 1994;372:672–676.

16 Shaikh MG, Boyes L, Kingston H, Collins R, Besley GT, Padmakumar B, Ismayl O, Hughes IA, Hall CM, Hellerud C, Achermann JC, Clayton PE: Skewed X inactivation is associated with phenotype in a female with adrenal hypoplasia congenital. J Med Genet 2008;45:e1–e5.

17 Takahashi T, Shoji Y, Shoji Y, Haraguchi N, Takahashi I, Takada G: Active hypothalamic-pituitary-gonadal axis in an infant with X-linked adrenal hypoplasia congenita. J Pediatr 1997;130: 485–488.

18 Tabarin A, Achermann JC, Recan D, Bex V, Bertagna X, Christin-Maitre S, Ito M, Jameson JL, Bouchard P: A novel mutation in DAX1 causes delayed-onset adrenal insufficiency and incomplete hypogonadotropic hypogonadism. J Clin Invest 2000;105:321–328.
19 Domenice S, Latronico AC, Brito VN, Arnhold IJP, Kok F, Mendonca BB: Adrenocorticotropin-dependent precocious puberty of testicular origin in a boy with x-linked adrenal hypoplasia congenita due to a novel mutation in the DAX1 gene. J Clin Endocrinol Metab 2001;86:4068–4071.
20 Montague CT, Farooqi IS, Whitehead JP, Soos MA, Rau H, Wareham NJ, Sewter CP, Digby JE, Mohammed SN, Hurst JA, Cheetham CH, Earley AR, Barnett AH, Prins JB, O'Rahilly S: Congenital leptin deficiency is associated with severe early-onset obesity in humans. Nature 1997;387:903–908.
21 Farooqi IS, Wangensteen T, Collins S, et al: Clinical and molecular genetic spectrum of congenital deficiency of the leptin receptor. N Engl J Med 2007;356:237–247.
22 Farooqi IS, Matarese G, Lord GM: Beneficial effects of leptin on obesity, T cell hyporesponsiveness, and neuroendocrine/metabolic dysfunction of human congenital leptin deficiency. J Clin Invest 2002;110:1093–1103.
23 Welt CK, Chan JL, Bullen J, Murphy R, Smith P, DePaoli AM, Karalis A, Mantzoros CS: Recombinant human leptin in women with hypothalamic amenorrhea. N Engl J Med 2004;351:987–997.
24 Jackson RS, Creemers JW, Ohagi S, Raffin-Sanson ML, Sanders L, Montague CT, Hutton JC, O'Rahilly S: Obesity and impaired prohormone processing associated with mutations in the human prohormone convertase 1 gene. Nat Genet 1997;16:303–306.
25 Jackson RS, Creemers JW, Farooqi IS, et al: Small-intestinal dysfunction accompanies the complex endocrinopathy of human proprotein convertase 1 deficiency. J Clin Invest 2003;112:1550–1560.
26 Farooqi IS, Volders K, Stanhope RG, Heuschkel R, White A, Lank E, Keogh J, O'Rahilly S, Creemers JW: Hyperphagia and early-onset obesity due to a novel homoxygous mutation in prohormone convertase 1/3. J Clin Endocrinol Metab 2007;92:3369–3373.
27 Zaghloul NA, Katsanis N: Mechanistic insights into Bardet-Biedl syndrome, a model ciliopathy. J Clin Invest 2009;119:428–437.
28 Harville HM, Held S, Diaz-Font A, Davis EE, Diplas BH, Lewis RA, Borochowitz ZU, Zhou W, Chaki M, Macdonald J, Kayserili H, Beales PL, Katsanis N, Otto E, Hildebrandt F: Identification of 11 novel mutations in 8 BBS genes by high-resolution homozygosity mapping. J Med Genet 2009, Epub ahead of print.

Dr. Timothy D. Cheetham
Department of Paediatric Endocrinology, Great North Children's Hospital
Royal Victoria Infirmary
Newcastle-upon-Tyne NE1 4LP (UK)
Tel. +44 191 2828562, Fax +44 191 2820306, E-Mail tim.cheetham@nuth.nhs.uk

Quinton R (ed): Kallmann Syndrome and Hypogonadotropic Hypogonadism.
Front Horm Res. Basel, Karger, 2010, vol 39, pp 168–169

Concluding Remarks

Balasubramanian Ravikumar · William F. Crowley, Jr.

Reproductive Endocrine Unit, Massachusetts General Hospital, Boston, Mass., USA

Ever since its first description, human gonadotropin-releasing hormone (GnRH) deficiency has been recognized both clinically and genetically as a heterogeneous disease. The growing appreciation that both Kallmann syndrome and normosmic idiopathic hypogonadotropic hypogonadism occur within a given family, i.e. with the same genetic milieu, demonstrates that both of these variants of GnRH deficiency are part of a continuous spectrum of clinical and genetic defects rather than single unique phenotypes. Those with anosmia signal a joint involvement of the olfactory system and GnRH neurons during their embryonic development, whereas those with a normal sense of smell indicate processes occurring either before or after migration of GnRH neurons.

Despite the critical evolutionary role played by the reproductive system in ensuring survival of the species, mammalian reproductive activity is quite remarkably invested in a single GnRH-encoding gene and a unique network of relatively sparse hypothalamic GnRH neurons. Considering the ever-changing environmental demands that have threatened survival of mammals over the millennia, it has been recognized that a multi-tiered, overlapping genetic network and cellular pathways must have evolved to regulate the secretion of GnRH itself. In keeping with this notion, the study of humans with GnRH deficiency and study of animal models of hypogonadotropic hypogonadism have been prismatic in unraveling the fascinating ontogeny of GnRH neurons, and the last decade has witnessed the discovery of a number of novel genes that underlie human GnRH deficiency.

An entire series of ligand-receptor pairs have now been linked to GnRH deficiency. As an evolving theme, mutations in the receptor are a dominant contributor to the syndrome compared to its cognate ligand(s). However, pathogenic genetic mutations account for only approximately a third of GnRH-deficient patients and, in many cases, mutations have been found in the heterozygous state, suggesting that a substantial number of genes underlying GnRH neuron ontogeny are yet to be discovered. In addition, there is an emerging evidence of oligogenicity and genotypic synergism in the pathogenesis of human GnRH deficiency, thus explaining the variable expressivity and incomplete penetrance seen within families with GnRH deficiency. Moreover, the spontaneous reversal of GnRH deficiency and the syndrome of adult-onset hypogonadotropic hypogonadism argue strongly in favor of significant gene-environment interactions and the potential role of hitherto unidentified modifier genes. The confluence of unique genetic variants in the pathogenesis of GnRH deficiency also highlights the significant prevalence of these mutant alleles among the general population. In fact, some PROKR2 variants are seen in various diverse populations, suggesting an ancient mutation, i.e. a common founder event, and even argue for the possibility of these variants contributing to a survival benefit and consequent positive natural selection in the population.

The growing genetic, clinical and molecular complexity of this human syndrome now warrants an integrated investigatory approach, encompassing detailed phenotyping of GnRH-deficient subjects, use of next generation gene sequencing to aid novel gene discovery and the use of bioinformatics to expand the biology of the evolving pathways. The precise biological basis for cessation of childhood and the onset of human puberty has been cited as one of the critical unanswered questions in the 21st century. The prismatic human model of GnRH deficiency presents us with a unique biologic opportunity to unravel the molecular basis of the arousal of the GnRH pulse generator to signal puberty in humans.

Prof. William F. Crowley, Jr.
Reproductive Endocrine Unit, Massachusetts General Hospital
55 Fruit Street
Boston, MA 02114 (USA)
Tel. +1 617 7263038, Fax +1 617 7265357, E-Mail wcrowley@partners.org

Author Index

Subject Index